Pediatric Reference Ranges

Third Edition

Edited by

Steven J. Soldin, PhD
Department of Laboratory Medicine
Children's National Medical Center
and George Washington University
School of Medicine
Washington, DC

Carlo Brugnara, MD
Department of Laboratory Medicine
Children's Hospital
and Harvard University
Boston, MA

Jocelyn M. Hicks, PhD
Department of Laboratory Medicine
Children's National Medical Center
and George Washington University
School of Medicine
Washington, DC

AACC Press
2101 L Street, NW, Suite 202
Washington, DC 20037-1526

ISBN 1-890883-22-0

Printed in the United States of America

We dedicate this book to our children and grandchildren.
We hope that children worldwide will benefit from this
third edition of *Pediatric Reference Ranges*.

FOREWORD

Pediatric Reference Ranges is now in its third edition. This invaluable volume on pediatric laboratory medicine is a very important contribution to patient care, now made even more useful by the addition of a greatly expanded chemistry section and more complete hematology reference ranges. Every children's hospital, pediatric department, and clinical laboratory should have this well-designed and easy-to-read manual close at hand. The authors are to be commended for their splendid addition to the quality of laboratory diagnosis.

David G. Nathan, M.D.
Dana Farber Cancer Institute
Boston, Massachusetts

Preface

Pediatric Reference Ranges:
Children are not Little Adults

Steven J. Soldin, PhD, FACB, FCACB

Children are unique individuals and not miniature adults. For example, neonates and premature infants have immature hepatic, renal, and pulmonary function. This affects the way these individuals handle drugs. Furthermore, their pediatric reference ranges for numerous analytes in many cases are clearly different from those found in older children and adults.

How drug metabolism changes with age
The majority of drugs are metabolized by the hepatic microsomal enzyme system, which is under genetic control and subject to many factors that influence its activity. If, for instance, patients eat char-broiled meat or inhale the smoke of cigarettes, the activity of the microsomal system is enhanced, increasing the clearance of the drug being given and shortening its half life. Such patients may require dosage adjustements. Age is another major influence. In the neonate, the hepatic microsomal enzyme systems and renal and hepatic function are immature. Therefore, a much smaller dose per kilo must be given to attain the same therapeutic concentration of a drug. During the first four months of life, infants need to be followed closely, because the enzyme activity is increasing, causing major changes in dosage requirement. In children from about four months of age to puberty, the hepatic microsomal enzyme system has approximately double the activity of the adult, requiring about double the dose per kilo to achieve the same therapeutic concentration as an adult.

As the youth goes through puberty, the activity of the system begins decreasing, and eventually the individual has essentially the same hepatic microsomal enzyme system activity as an adult. One has to monitor closely if he/she is on drug therapy and going through puberty, because the activity of the enzyme system is changing a great deal over that time period.

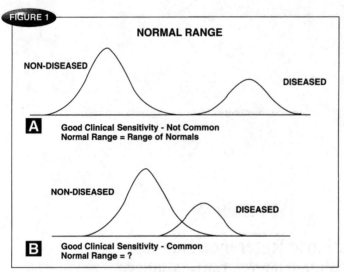

Fig.1: Normal range plots for two analytes.

The concept of reference ranges

In order to determine if a patient suffers from a particular disease, clinicians will order tests that will confirm or refute their suspicions. A laboratory test is often the starting point for the differential diagnosis of a particular disease from among a spectrum of possible diseases. There are many different ways to establish age- and sex-related reference values, each method with its own inherent advantages and disadvantages. These include obtaining specimens from known "healthy" individuals and after removing the extreme outliers, tabulating values from the lowest to highest and removing the 0-2.5[th] percentile and the 97.5-100.00[th] percentile, thereby leaving a range of the 2.5-97.5[th] percentile for any particular anlayte. One can also use the mean ± standard deviation (SD) approach, but for this method to be valid, the frequency distribution of values must be Gaussian (symmetrical or bell-shaped distribution). If the data are skewed and non-Gaussian, it can often be made Gaussian by plotting the log of the value instead of the value itself. Once a Gaussian distribution is obtained, one can calculate the reference range from the mean ± 2 SD.

Fig. 1 shows normal range plots for two different analytes. In (A) there is no overlap between the diseased and nondiseased populations. An example may be urinary vanillymandelic acid (VMA) or homovanillic acid (HVA) often ordered to confirm a diagnosis of pheochromocytoma or neuroblastoma. In (B), there is some overlap between the diseased and nondiseased populations. This situation is more common and choosing the normal reference range cut-off point here is somewhat arbitrary. In general, most clinicians are acquainted with a range that encompasses the 2.5-97.5[th] percentile of the population.

Hoffmann's approach to determining reference ranges

A third approach is to use the results obtained from hospitalized sick patients to develop the normal reference intervals. While this may seem to be a strange approach it has many advantages, especially in developing reference ranges for children. It is almost impossible to obtain a large enough population of healthy children between the ages of 1 day and 18 years who are prepared to donate blood specimens, or to obtain the informed consent necessary thereby allowing reference range studies to be performed.[1] By using either Chauvenet's or Dixon's criteria for removing outliers and then plotting % cumulative frequency versus the laboratory value (or log of the value, if non-Gaussian distribution), one obtains a straight line, which deviates from linearity at both ends. This straight line can be extended to provide the 2.5[th] and 97.5[th] percentiles for the population being studied. This approach has been described in detail by Hoffmann,[2] and an example for glucose is shown in Fig. 2. This approach, apart from its simplicity and appeal in pediatrics, has additional advantages for analytes such as T_4 (thyroxine) and cholesterol. T_4 values are significantly increased in a "sick" population. To assess the thyroid function in the "sick" population and differentiate those patients with thyroid disease from those with other ailments, it makes eminent sense to know the T_4 reference intervals for the "sick" population. Values above or below the 2.5[th]-97.5[th] range would then indicate the distinct possibility of thyroid disease. The same is true for cholesterol, values of which decrease somewhat in a "sick population."

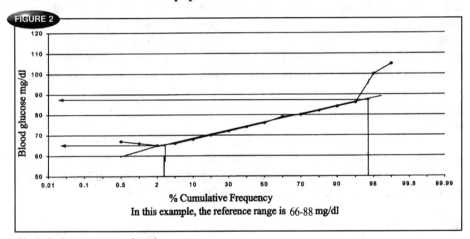

FIGURE 2

In this example, the reference range is 66-88 mg/dl

Fig.2: Reference range for glucose.

Reference ranges are method-dependent
It is important to emphasize that reference ranges vary with the method (technology) used to measure the analytes in question. In compiling the pediatric reference ranges for a text-book, I could not help noticing the very large differences one found for many endocrine tests, even if the same patient samples were used to establish these ranges. For example, when analyzing T_4, the male 1-30 day ranges using the Abbott IMx are 3.0-14.4 ug/dL (39-185 nmol/L) while the T_4 Gamma Coat (Baxter-Travenol Diagnostics, Cambridge, MA, USA) results are 5.9-21.5 ug/dL (76-276 nmol/l).[3] Such differences are extraordinary and indicate the considerable nonspecificity of antibodies used in immunoassays in the mid to late 1990's. One may well ask, what are we really measuring?

Children are not "little adults"
The reference ranges for many analytes vary significantly from birth through the end

of puberty, as already stated. Neonates (and premature neonates), for example, have immature hepatic, renal, and pulmonary function. The normal values for blood gases, therefore, differ significantly from those of older children (pH 7.18-7.51 versus 7.35-7.44, respectively). The same is true for electrolytes such as Na+, K+, Ca++, where reference ranges are somewhat broader than those found later in life. For example, for ionized calcium, the reference range for 0-1 month babies is 3.9-6.0 mg/dL (1.0-1.5 mmol/L) while in the adult it is 4.7-5.3 mg/dL (1.18-1.32 mmol/L)

Reference ranges for many enzymes vary significantly with age. For example, on the Vitros analyzer (Johnson & Johnson, Rochester, NY, USA) the male and female 97.5[th] percentile ranges for amylase are 30, 50, 80 and 100 U/L for 0-0.2, 0.2-0.5, 0.5-1.0, and 1-19 years, respectively. For aspartate aminotransferase (AST, SGOT), the male 2.5-97.5[th] percentiles using the Vitros analyzer are 30-100, 20-70, 15-45 U/L for 1-7 days, 8-30 days and 16-19 years, respectively.

Values for many endocrine tests undergo significant changes with onset of puberty. Male and female ranges can, and often do, differ significantly. In order to aid clinicians and pediatricians in interpreting laboratory data, we have recently gathered the literature available in this area, and published it in this textbook, Pediatric Reference Ranges. This book provides the reference ranges on a wide variety of analytes for children (males and females) from neonates to adolescents and young adults.[3]

Conclusion
Anyone who uses reference ranges should realize that they are guidelines for the clinician and cannot be used as definitive indicators of health or pathologic states. Values for healthy and diseased individuals can overlap, and significant inter- and intra-individual differences exist even among healthy individuals.[3]

References
1. Soldin SJ, Rifai N, Hicks JM (eds): Biochemical Basis of Pediatric Disease (3rd ed), Washington DC, USA, AACC Press, 1998.
2. Hoffmann RG: Statistics in the practice of medicine. JAMA 1963; 185:864-73).
3. Soldin SJ, Brugnara SJ, Hicks, JM. (eds): Pediatric Reference Ranges (3rd ed), Washington DC, USA, AACC Press, 1999.

INTRODUCTION

This book provides reference (normal) ranges on a wide variety of analytes for children from neonates to adolescents and young adults. We have put the emphasis on a user-friendly format. Each page has the same layout and provides information on the reference to the study. Wherever possible, the work is our own or from the very recent literature. The type of fluid analyzed is given along with the methodology. We have tried to include at least two references for each analyte. We have quoted the different methodologies used. The names of the tests are reported alphabetically, and alternate names are sometimes given. In our studies, we have used a large number (*n*) of children in each age group, generally between 50 and 100. The reference values are reported by age and sex, and wherever possible we have included SI units so that this book can be used throughout the world. We have included the statistical basis by which the reference ranges were calculated and the population source.

We have purposely not burdened this book with clinical information that can be found elsewhere, especially in our previous book entitled *The Biochemical Basis of Pediatric Disease*, which we co-edited with Dr. Nader Rifai. It is our belief that, for the most part, when a physician or laboratory scientist seeks information about reference ranges, that is all he or she is interested in!

Anyone who uses reference ranges should realize that they are guidelines for the clinician and cannot be used as definitive indicators of health or pathological states. Values for healthy and diseased individuals often overlap, and, more importantly, considerable variations exist even among healthy individuals. Values also can vary according to the methodology used.

This book would not have been possible without the enormous help from American Medical Laboratories, Inc.® in Chantilly, Virginia. They provided the analyses for many of our studies as well as the complex statistical assistance that was necessary since our data was derived from patients of our hospital. In particular, our heartfelt thanks go to Dr. Ira D. Godwin and Dr. C. Barrie Cook for making the funding available, and to Mr. Jimmy Bailey, Ms. Jan Beatey, Ms. Susan Bjorn, Ms. Pam Watson, and Mr. James Cook for their invaluable assistance.

Steven J. Soldin
Carlo Brugnara
Jocelyn M. Hicks

CONTENTS

Amino Acids (Plasma) *Continued*

Amino Acids (Urine) 21

Amino Acids (Urine) *Continued*

Chemistry Tests

ALANINE AMINOTRANSFERASE
(ALT, SGPT)

Test	Age	Male		Female	
		n	U/L	n	U/L
1.	1 - 7d	109	6 - 40	84	7 - 40
	8 - 30d	168	10 - 40	71	8 - 32
	1 - 3mo	178	13 - 39	173	12 - 47
	4 - 6mo	135	12 - 42	59	12 - 37
	7 - 12mo	130	13 - 45	107	12 - 41
2.	1 - 3y	50*	5 - 45	50*	5 - 45
	4 - 6y	40*	10 - 25	40*	10 - 25
	7 - 9y	80*	10 - 35	80*	10 - 35
	10 - 11y	27	10 - 35	34	10 - 30
	12 - 13y	31	10 - 55	49	10 - 30
	14 - 15y	26	10 - 45	52	5 - 30
	16 - 19y	40	10 - 40	61	5 - 35
3.	1 - 30d	50	1 - 25	51	2 - 25
	31 - 365d	91	4 - 35	76	3 - 30
	1 - 3y	119	5 - 30	115	5 - 30
	4 - 6y	114	5 - 20	101	5 - 25
	7 - 9y	102	5 - 25	109	5 - 25
	10 - 18y	280	5 - 30	269	5 - 20

Specimen Type: 1,2,3 Plasma, Serum

Reference:

1. Soldin SJ, Savwoir TV, Guo Y. Pediatric reference ranges for alkaline phosphatase, aspartate aminotransferase, and alanine aminotransferase in children less than 1 year old on the Vitros 500. Clin Chem 1997;43:S199. (Abstract)

2. Lockitch G, Halstead AC, Albersheim S, et al. Age and sex specific pediatric reference intervals for biochemistry analytes as measured with the Ektachem 700 analyzer. Clin Chem 1988;34:1622-5.

3. Soldin SJ, Bailey J, Bjorn S, et al. Pediatric reference ranges for ALT. Clin Chem 1995;41:S92-3. (Abstract)

Method(s):

1, 2 Ektachem 500 (1) and 700 (2) (Johnson & Johnson, Rochester, NY).

3. Measured on the Hitachi 747 using Boehringer-Mannheim reagents. (Boehringer-Mannheim Diagnostics, Indianapolis, IN.)

Comments:

1, 3 Study used hospitalized patients and a computerized approach adapted from the Hoffmann technique to obtain the 2.5 - 97.5th percentiles.

2. The study population was healthy children. Non-parametric methods were used to determine the 0.025 and 0.975 fractiles.

*No significant differences were found for males and females. These ranges were therefore derived from combined data.

ALBUMIN

Test	Age	Male n	Male g/dL	Male g/L	Female n	Female g/dL	Female g/L
1.	1 - 7d	161	2.3 - 3.8	23 - 38	132	1.8 - 3.9	18 – 39
	8 - 30d	252	2.0 – 4.5	20 - 45	124	1.8 – 4.4	18 - 44
	31 – 90d	199	2.0 - 4.8	20 - 48	178	1.9 – 4.2	19 – 42
	91 – 180d	135	2.1 – 4.9	21 - 49	121	2.2 – 4.4	22 - 44
	181d – 1y	295	2.1 – 4.7	21 - 47	267	2.2 – 4.7	22 - 47
2.	0 - 5d (< 2.5 kg)	30	2.0 - 3.6	20 - 36	30	2.0 - 3.6	20 - 36
	0 - 5d (> 2.5 kg)	93	2.6 - 3.6	26 - 36	93	2.6 - 3.6	26 - 36
	1 - 3y	50	3.4 - 4.2	34 - 42	50	3.4 - 4.2	34 - 42
	4 - 6y	38	3.5 - 5.2	35 - 52	38	3.5 - 5.2	35 - 52
	7 - 9y	74	3.7 - 5.6	37 - 56	74	3.7 - 5.6	37 - 56
	10 - 19y	332	3.7 - 5.6	37 - 56	332	3.7 - 5.6	37 - 56
3.	1 - 30d	73	2.6 - 4.1	26 - 41	51	2.7 - 4.3	27 - 43
	31 - 182d	58	2.8 - 4.6	28 - 46	30	2.9 - 4.2	29 - 42
	183 - 365d	29	2.8 - 4.8	28 - 48	42	3.3 - 4.8	33 - 48
	1 - 18y	652	3.2 - 4.7	32 - 47	626	2.9 - 4.2	29 - 42

Specimen Type:	1, 2, 3 Plasma, Serum
Reference:	1. Soldin SJ, Morse AS. Pediatric reference ranges for Albumin and Total Protein in Children <1 Year Old using the Vitros 500 Analyzer. Clin Chem 1998;44:A15. (Abstract) 2. Lockitch G, Halstead AC, Albersheim S, et al. Age and sex specific pediatric reference intervals for biochemistry analytes as measured with the Ektachem 700 analyzer. Clin Chem 1988;34:1622-5. 3. Soldin SJ, Bjorn S, Beatey J, et al. Pediatric reference ranges for albumin, globulin and total protein on the Hitachi 747. Clin Chem 1995;41:S93. (Abstract)
Method(s):	1. Bromocresol green method. Ektachem 500 (Johnson & Johnson, Rochester, NY). 2. Bromocresol green method. Ektachem 700 (Johnson & Johnson, Rochester, NY). 3. Boehringer-Mannheim albumin reagent (bromocresol green). Albumin was measured on the Hitachi 747 (Boehringer-Mannheim Diagnostics, Indianapolis, IN).
Comments:	1, 3 Study used hospitalized patients and a computerized approach adapted from the Hoffmann technique. Values are 2.5 - 97.5 percentiles. 2. Healthy normal children. Values are 2.5 - 97.5 percentiles.

ALDOLASE

Age	n	Male and Female U/L
10 - 24mo	40	3.4 - 11.8
25mo - 16y	23	1.2 - 8.8
17 - 64y	30	1.7 - 4.9

Specimen Type:	Serum
Reference:	Visnapuu LA, Karlson LK, Dubinsky EH, et al. Pediatric reference ranges for serum aldolase. Am J Clin Pathol 1989;91:476-7.
Method(s):	Aldolase Test Stat Pak (Behring Diagnostics, La Jolla, CA).
Comments:	Essentially healthy children and adults were used in the study. Results are mean ± 2SD.

ALDOSTERONE

Test	Age	n	Male and Female	
			ng/dL	pmol/L
1.	6 – 9y	25	1 - 24	28 - 666
	10 – 11y	23	2 - 15	55 - 416
	12 – 14y	27	1 - 22	28 - 610
	15 – 17y	42	1 - 32	28 - 888
2.	<1y	*	5.8 - 110	160 – 3000
	1 – <4y	*	2.5 - 36	70 – 1000
	4 – <10y (P_1)	*	1 - 22	30 – 600
	P_2	*	1.5 – 22	40 – 600
	P_3	*	1.5 – 22	40 – 600
	P_4	*	1.5 – 22	40 – 600
	P_5	*	1.5 – 22	40 – 600

Specimen Type:	1.	Serum
	2.	Serum/Plasma
Reference:	1.	Nichols Institute. Pediatric endocrine testing, 1993:1.
	2.	Biochemical Basis of Pediatric Disease, Eds. Soldin SJ, Rifai N, Hicks JM. 3rd Edition 1998 AACC Press. Chapter 9 'Disorders of the Adrenal Gland' p 233.
Method(s):	1.	Extraction, chromatography. Radioimmunoassay.
	2.	See reference.
Comments:	1.	Upright posture, normal sodium diet. Results are 2.5 - 97.5th percentiles.
	2.	These reference ranges are for guidance only. Numbers not provided. $P_1 – P_5$ refer to pubertal stages.

ALKALINE PHOSPHATASE (ALP)

Test	Age	Male n	Male U/L	Female n	Female U/L
1.	1 – 7d	141	77 - 265	109	65 - 270
	8 – 30d	203	91 - 375	141	65 - 365
	1 - 3mo	251	60 - 360	234	80 - 425
	4 - 6mo	129	55 - 325	66	80 - 345
	7 – 12mo	113	60 - 300	58	60 - 330
2.**	1 – 3y	50*	129 – 291	50*	129 – 291
	4 – 6y	40*	134 – 346	40*	134 – 346
	7 – 9y	80*	156 – 386	80*	156 – 386
	10 – 11y	27	120 – 488	34	116 – 515
	12 – 13y	31	178 – 455	49	93 – 386
	14 – 15y	26	116 – 483	52	62 – 209
	16 – 19y	40	58 – 237	61	45 – 116
3.	1 – 30d	60	75 - 316	75	48 - 406
	31 – 365d	132	82 - 383	122	124 - 341
	1 – 3y	136	104 - 345	111	108 - 317
	4 - 6y	113	93 - 309	113	96 - 297
	7 - 9y	124	86 - 315	104	69 - 325
	10 – 12y	111	42 - 362	109	51 - 332
	13 - 15y	126	74 - 390	105	50 - 162
	16 - 18y	112	52 - 171	110	47 - 119

Specimen Type:	1, 3	Plasma, Serum
	2.	Serum
Reference:	1.	Soldin SJ, Savwoir TV, Guo Y. Pediatric reference ranges for alkaline phosphatase, aspartate aminotransferase, and alanine aminotransferase in children less than 1 year old on the Vitros 500. Clin Chem 1997;43:S199. (Abstract)
	2.	Lockitch G, Halstead AC, Albersheim S, et al. Age and sex specific pediatric reference intervals for biochemistry analytes as measured with the Ektachem 700 analyzer. Clin Chem 1988;34:1622-5.
	3.	Soldin SJ, Hicks JM, Bailey J, et al. Pediatric reference ranges for alkaline phosphatase on the Hitachi 747 analyzer. 1997;43:S198. (Abstract)
Method(s):	1, 2	Ektachem 500 and 700 (Johnson & Johnson, Rochester, NY). p-Nitrophenylphosphate.
	3.	Hitachi 747. Boehringer-Mannheim reagents (p-Nitrophenylphosphate). (Boehringer-Mannheim Diagnostics, Indianapolis, IN.)
Comments:	1, 3	Study used hospitalized patients and a computerized approach adapted from the Hoffmann technique to obtain the 2.5 - 97.5th percentiles.
	2.	The study population was healthy children. Non-parametric methods were used to determine the 0.025 and 0.975 fractiles. *No significant differences were found for males and females. These ranges were therefore derived from combined data. ** Due to changes made by the manufacturer in slide performance, these results are lower than those published by the author.

ALPHA₁-ANTITRYPSIN
(α_1-AT)

Test	Age	Male			Female		
		n	mg/dL	g/L	n	mg/dL	g/L
1.	0 - 5d	73*	143 - 440	1.43 - 4.40	73*	143 - 440	1.43 - 4.40
	1 - 3y	51*	147 - 244	1.47 - 2.44	51*	147 - 244	1.47 - 2.44
	4 - 6y	39*	160 - 245	1.60 - 2.45	39*	160 - 245	1.60 - 2.45
	7 - 9y	39*	160 - 245	1.60 - 2.45	39*	160 - 245	1.60 - 2.45
	10 - 13y	36	162 - 249	1.62 - 2.49	45	166 - 267	1.66 - 2.67
	14 - 19y	46	152 - 317	1.52 - 3.17	66	176 - 298	1.76 - 2.98

Test	Age	Male and Female		
		n	mg/dL	g/L
2.	0 - 1mo	60	124 - 348	1.24 - 3.48
	1 - 6mo	45	111 - 297	1.11 - 2.97
	6mo - 2y	82	95 - 251	0.95 - 2.51
	2 - 19y	303	110 - 279	1.10 - 2.79

Specimen Type:	1, 2 Serum
Reference:	1. Lockitch G, Halstead AC, Quigley G, et al. Age and sex specific pediatric reference intervals: study design and methods illustrated by measurement of serum proteins with the Behring LN Nephelometer. Clin Chem 1988;34:1618-21.
	2. Davis ML, Austin C, Messmer BL, et al. IFCC-standardized pediatric reference intervals for 10 serum proteins using Beckman Array 360 system. Clin Biochem 1996;29:489-92.
Method(s):	1. Nephelometric with Behring LN nephelometer (Behring Diagnostics, Hoechst Canada, Inc., Montreal).
	2. Beckman Array 360 (Beckman Instruments, Brea CA)
Comments:	1. Normal healthy children. This data set excluded children found to have SZ, MZ, or ZZ phenotypes by protease inhibitor typing.
	Note: Type MM = normal; Type MS = normal variant (~ 8% of population); MZ = heterozygous for deficiency (< 2% of population). ZZ = homozygous for deficiency. PI typing necessary if result is low. Since α_1-AT is an acute phase reactant, MZ individuals may have normal values. Values are 2.5 - 97.5th percentiles.
	*Results from males and females combined. Values provided are 0.025 - 0.975 fractiles.
	2. Samples were obtained from children attending outpatient clinics. Results are 2.5 - 97.5th percentiles.

ALPHA-FETOPROTEIN

Test	Age	Males		Non-Pregnant Females	
		n	ng/mL µg/L	n	ng/mL µg/L
1.	0 - 1mo	71	0.6 - 16387	58	0.6 - 18964
	1 - 12mo	113	0.6 - 28.3	102	0.6 - 77.0
	1 - 3y	134	0.6 - 7.9	116	0.6 - 11.1
	4 - 6y	101	0.6 - 5.6	118	0.6 - 4.2
	7 - 12y	138	0.6 - 3.7	120	0.6 - 5.6
	13 - 18y	145	0.6 - 3.9	122	0.6 - 4.2
2.	Birth	*	Very High	*	Very High
	Adult	*	< 5	*	< 5

Specimen Type:	1, 2	Plasma
Reference:	1.	Soldin SJ, Hicks JM, Godwin ID, et al. Pediatric reference ranges for alpha-fetoprotein. Clin Chem 1992;38:959. (Abstract)
	2.	Reference values and S.I. Unit Information. The Hospital for Sick Children, Toronto, Canada 1993:355.
Method(s):	1, 2	Abbott EIA procedure. (Abbott Laboratories, Abbott Park, IL.)
Comments:	1.	Study used hospitalized patients and a computerized adaptation of the Hoffmann technique. Values are 2.5 - 97.5 percentiles.
	2.	Also increased during rapid liver regeneration, eg., after acute hepatitis.
		*Information not given in the reference.

AMINO ACIDS (PLASMA)

Test	Age	n	Male and Female nmol/mL			
			Alanine	β-alanine	Anserine	α-amino-adipic acid
1.	Premature (first 6 wk)	*	212 - 504	0	--	0
	0 - 1mo	*	131 - 710	0 - 10	0	0
	1 - 24mo	*	143 - 439	0 - 7	0	0
	2 - 18y	*	152 - 547	0 - 7	0	0
	Adult	*	177 - 583	0 - 12	0	0 - 6
2.	6mo	*	182 - 396	--	--	--
	2y	*	173 - 349	--	--	--
	6y	*	182 – 319	--	--	--
	16y	*	240 - 482	--	--	--

Specimen Type:	1,2 Plasma
Reference:	1. Shapira E, Blitzer MG, Miller JB, Africk DK, Eds. Biochemical genetics: A laboratory manual. Oxford, UK: Oxford University Press, 1989;94-5. 2. Lepage N, McDonald N, Dallaire L, et al. Age-Specific distribution of plasma amino acid concentrations in a healthy pediatric population. Clin Chem 1997; 43: 2397-2402
Method(s):	1. Beckman amino-acid analyzer. Beckman 6300 (Beckman Instruments Inc., Palo Alto, CA). 2. Beckman amino-acid analyzer. Beckman 7300 (Beckman Instruments Inc., Palo Alto, CA).
Comments:	1. Results are mean ± 2SD. 2. Results are 10 – 90th percentiles in healthy children. *See reference for numbers.

AMINO ACIDS (PLASMA)

Test	Age	n	α-amino-n-butyric acid	γ-amino-butyric acid	β-amino-isobutyric acid	Arginine
			Male and Female nmol/mL			
1.	Premature (first 6 wk)	*	14 - 52	0	0	34 - 96
	0 - 1mo	*	8 - 24	0 - 2	0	6 - 140
	1 - 24mo	*	3 - 26	0	0	12 - 133
	2 - 18y	*	4 - 31	0	0	10 - 140
	Adult	*	5 - 41	0	0	15 - 128
2.	6mo	*	--	--	--	43 - 120
	2y	*	--	--	--	46 - 90
	6y	*	--	--	--	50 - 99
	16y	*	--	--	--	68 - 128

Specimen Type:	1,2 Plasma
Reference:	1. Shapira E, Blitzer MG, Miller JB, Africk DK, Eds. Biochemical genetics: A laboratory manual. Oxford, UK: Oxford University Press, 1989:94-5. 2. Lepage N, McDonald N, Dallaire L, et al. Age-Specific distribution of plasma amino acid concentrations in a healthy pediatric population. Clin Chem 1997; 43: 2397-2402
Method(s):	1. Beckman amino-acid analyzer. Beckman 6300 (Beckman Instruments Inc., Palo Alto, CA). 2. Beckman amino-acid analyzer. Beckman 7300 (Beckman Instruments Inc., Palo Alto, CA).
Comments:	1. Results are mean ± 2SD. 2. Results are 10 – 90th percentiles in healthy children. *See reference for numbers.

12

AMINO ACIDS (PLASMA)

Test	Age	n	Male and Female nmol/mL			
			Asparagine	Aspartic acid	Carnosine	Citrulline
1.	Premature (first 6 wk)	*	90 - 295	24 - 50	- -	20 - 87
	0 - 1mo	*	29 - 132	20 - 129	0 - 19	10 - 45
	1 - 24mo	*	21 - 95	0 - 23	0	3 - 35
	2 - 18y	*	23 - 112	1 - 24	0	1 - 46
	Adult	*	35 - 74	1 - 25	0	12 - 55
2.	6mo	*	31 - 56	4 - 18	- -	14 - 32
	2y	*	29 - 56	3 - 8	- -	17 - 35
	6y	*	31 - 67	3 - 6	- -	23 - 37
	16y	*	37 - 81	2 - 5	- -	23 - 39

Specimen Type:	1,2 Plasma
Reference:	1. Shapira E, Blitzer MG, Miller JB, Africk DK, Eds. Biochemical genetics: a laboratory manual. Oxford, UK: Oxford University Press, 1989:94-5. 2. Lepage N, McDonald N, Dallaire L, et al. Age-Specific distribution of plasma amino acid concentrations in a healthy pediatric population. Clin Chem 1997; 43: 2397-402
Method(s):	1. Beckman amino-acid analyzer. Beckman 6300 (Beckman Instruments Inc., Palo Alto, CA). 2. Beckman amino-acid analyzer. Beckman 7300 (Beckman Instruments Inc., Palo Alto, CA).
Comments:	1. Results are mean ± 2SD. 2. Results are 10 – 90th percentiles in healthy children. *See reference for numbers.

AMINO ACIDS (PLASMA)

Test	Age	n	Cystathionine	Cystine	Ethanolamine	Glutamic Acid
				Male and Female **nmol/mL**		
1.	Premature (first 6 wk)	*	5 - 10	15 - 70	--	107 - 276
	0 - 1mo	*	0 - 3	17 - 98	0 - 115	62 - 620
	1 - 24mo	*	0 - 5	16 - 84	0 - 4	10 - 133
	2 - 18y	*	0 - 3	5 - 45	0 - 7	5 - 150
	Adult	*	0 - 3	5 - 82	0 - 153	10 - 131
2.	6mo	*	--	21 - 53	--	31 - 113
	2y	*	--	27 - 52	--	28 - 81
	6y	*	--	33 - 54	--	13 - 65
	16y	*	--	36 - 61	--	11 - 46

Specimen Type:	1,2 Plasma
Reference:	1. Shapira E, Blitzer MG, Miller JB, Africk DK, Eds. Biochemical genetics: a laboratory manual. Oxford, UK: Oxford University Press, 1989:94-5. 2. Lepage N, McDonald N, Dallaire L, et al. Age-Specific distribution of plasma amino acid concentrations in a healthy pediatric population. Clin Chem 1997; 43: 2397-402
Method(s):	1. Beckman amino-acid analyzer. Beckman 6300 (Beckman Instruments Inc., Palo Alto, CA). 2. Beckman amino-acid analyzer. Beckman 7300 (Beckman Instruments Inc., Palo Alto, CA).
Comments:	1. Results are mean ± 2SD. 2. Results are 10 – 90th percentiles in healthy children. *See reference for numbers.

AMINO ACIDS (PLASMA)

Test	Age	n	Male and Female nmol/mL			
			Glutamine	Glycine	Histidine	Homocystine
1.	Premature (first 6 wk)	*	248 - 850	298 - 602	72 - 134	3 - 20
	0 - 1mo	*	376 - 709	232 - 740	30 - 138	0
	1 - 24mo	*	246 - 1,182	81 - 436	41 - 101	0
	2 - 18y	*	254 - 823	127 - 341	41 - 125	0 - 5
	Adult	*	205 - 756	151 - 490	72 - 124	0
2.	6mo	*	474 - 737	138 - 276	61 - 91	--
	2y	*	473 - 692	138 - 276	61 - 91	--
	6y	*	493 - 724	144 - 282	63 - 93	--
	16y	*	551 - 797	183 - 322	77 - 107	--

Specimen Type:	1,2 Plasma
Reference:	1. Shapira E, Blitzer MG, Miller JB, Africk DK, Eds. Biochemical genetics: A laboratory manual. Oxford, UK: Oxford University Press, 1989:94-5. 2. Lepage N, McDonald N, Dallaire L, et al. Age-Specific distribution of plasma amino acid concentrations in a healthy pediatric population. Clin Chem 1997; 43: 2397-402
Method(s):	1. Beckman amino-acid analyzer. Beckman 6300 (Beckman Instruments Inc., Palo Alto, CA). 2. Beckman amino-acid analyzer. Beckman 7300 (Beckman Instruments Inc., Palo Alto, CA).
Comments:	1. Results are mean ± 2SD. 2. Results are 10 –90th percentiles in healthy children. *See reference for numbers.

AMINO ACIDS (PLASMA)

Test	Age	n	Male and Female nmol/mL			
			Hydroxylysine	Hydroxyproline	Isoleucine	Leucine
1.	Premature (first 6 wk)	*	0	0 - 80	23 - 85	151 - 220
	0 - 1mo	*	0 - 7	0 - 91	26 - 91	48 - 160
	1 - 24mo	*	0 - 7	0 - 63	31 - 86	47 - 155
	2 - 18y	*	0 - 2	3 - 45	22 - 107	49 - 216
	Adult	*	0	0 - 53	30 - 108	72 - 201
2.	6mo	*	--	--	39 – 76	77 – 153
	2y	*	--	--	4 - 78	79 - 147
	6y	*	--	--	40 – 69	86 – 136
	16y	*	--	--	47 - 74	101 - 159

Specimen Type:	1,2 Plasma
Reference:	1. Shapira E, Blitzer MG, Miller JB, Africk DK, Eds. Biochemical genetics: a laboratory manual. Oxford, UK: Oxford University Press, 1989:94-5. 2. Lepage N, McDonald N, Dallaire L, et al. Age-Specific distribution of plasma amino acid concentrations in a healthy pediatric population. Clin Chem 1997; 43: 2397-402
Method(s):	1. Beckman amino-acid analyzer. Beckman 6300 (Beckman Instruments Inc., Palo Alto, CA). 2. Beckman amino-acid analyzer. Beckman 7300 (Beckman Instruments Inc., Palo Alto, CA).
Comments:	1. Results are mean ± 2SD. 2. Results are 10 –90th percentiles in healthy children. *See reference for numbers.

AMINO ACIDS (PLASMA)

Test	Age	n	Lysine	Methionine	1-Methyl-histidine	3-Methyl-histidine
			Male and Female nmol/mL			
1.	Premature (first 6 wk)	*	128 - 255	37 - 91	4 - 28	5 - 33
	0 - 1mo	*	92 - 325	10 - 60	0 - 43	0 - 5
	1 - 24mo	*	52 - 196	9 - 42	0 - 44	0 - 5
	2 - 18y	*	48 - 284	7 - 47	0 - 42	0 - 5
	Adult	*	116 - 296	10 - 42	0 - 39	0 - 8
2.	6mo	*	87 - 171	14 – 38	--	--
	2y	*	88 – 172	13 - 22	--	--
	6y	*	96 - 181	14 – 25	--	--
	16y	*	157 - 242	20 - 34	--	--

Specimen Type:	1,2 Plasma
Reference:	1. Shapira E, Blitzer MG, Miller JB, Africk DK, Eds. Biochemical genetics: a laboratory manual. Oxford, UK: Oxford University Press, 1989:94-5.
	2. Lepage N, McDonald N, Dallaire L, et al. Age-Specific distribution of plasma amino acid concentrations in a healthy pediatric population. Clin Chem 1997; 43: 2397-402
Method(s):	1. Beckman amino-acid analyzer. Beckman 6300 (Beckman Instruments Inc., Palo Alto, CA).
	2. Beckman amino-acid analyzer. Beckman 7300 (Beckman Instruments Inc., Palo Alto, CA).
Comments:	1. Results are mean ± 2SD.
	2. Results are 10 – 90th percentiles in healthy children.
	*See reference for numbers.

AMINO ACIDS (PLASMA)

Test	Age	n	Ornithine	Phenylalanine	Phospho-ethanolamine	Phospho- serine
				Male and Female **nmol/mL**		
1.	Premature (first 6 wk)	*	77 - 212	98 - 213	5 - 35	10 - 45
	0 - 1mo	*	48 - 211	38 - 137	3 - 27	7 - 47
	1 - 24mo	*	22 - 103	31 - 75	0 - 6	1 - 20
	2 - 18y	*	10 - 163	26 - 91	0 - 69	1 - 30
	Adult	*	48 - 195	35 - 85	0 - 40	2 - 14
2.	6mo	*	25 - 103	38 - 78	--	--
	2y	*	24 – 60	39 – 65	--	--
	6y	*	25 - 50	40 - 61	--	--
	16y	*	37 - 62	47 - 74	--	--

Specimen Type:	1,2 Plasma
Reference:	1. Shapira E, Blitzer MG, Miller JB, Africk DK, Eds. Biochemical genetics: a laboratory manual. Oxford, UK: Oxford University Press, 1989:94-5. 2. Lepage N, McDonald N, Dallaire L, et al. Age-Specific distribution of plasma amino acid concentrations in a healthy pediatric population. Clin Chem 1997; 43: 2397-402
Method(s):	1. Beckman amino-acid analyzer. Beckman 6300 (Beckman Instruments Inc., Palo Alto, CA). 2. Beckman amino-acid analyzer. Beckman 7300 (Beckman Instruments Inc., Palo Alto, CA).
Comments:	1. Results are mean ± 2SD. 2. Results are 10 – 90th percentiles in healthy children. *See reference for numbers.

AMINO ACIDS (PLASMA)

Test	Age	n	Male and Female nmol/mL			
			Proline	**Sarcosine**	**Serine**	**Taurine**
1.	Premature (first 6 wk)	*	92 - 310	0	127 - 248	151 - 411
	0 - 1mo	*	110 - 417	0 - 625	99 - 395	46 - 492
	1 - 24mo	*	52 - 298	0	71 - 186	15 - 143
	2 - 18y	*	59 - 369	0 - 9	69 - 187	10 - 170
	Adult	*	97 - 329	0	58 - 181	54 - 210
2.	6mo	*	93 - 265	--	98 - 160	39 – 111
	2y	*	93 – 220	--	97 - 154	39 - 80
	6y	*	93 - 201	--	96 - 155	41 - 69
	16y	*	113 - 271	--	101 - 177	41 - 66

Specimen Type:	1,2 Plasma
Reference:	1. Shapira E, Blitzer MG, Miller JB, Africk DK, Eds. Biochemical genetics: a laboratory manual. Oxford, UK: Oxford University Press, 1989:94-5. 2. Lepage N, McDonald N, Dallaire L, et al. Age-Specific distribution of plasma amino acid concentrations in a healthy pediatric population. Clin Chem 1997; 43: 2397-402
Method(s):	1. Beckman amino-acid analyzer. Beckman 6300 (Beckman Instruments Inc., Palo Alto, CA). 2. Beckman amino-acid analyzer. Beckman 7300 (Beckman Instruments Inc., Palo Alto, CA).
Comments:	1. Results are mean ± 2SD. 2. Results are 10 – 90th percentiles in healthy children. *See reference for numbers.

AMINO ACIDS (PLASMA)

Test	Age	n	Male and Female nmol/mL			
			Threonine	**Tryptophan**	**Tyrosine**	**Valine**
1.	Premature (first 6 wk)	*	150 - 330	28 - 136	147 - 420	99 - 220
	0 - 1mo	*	90 - 329	0 - 60	55 - 147	86 - 190
	1 - 24mo	*	24 - 174	23 - 71	22 - 108	64 - 294
	2 - 18y	*	35 - 226	0 - 79	24 - 115	74 - 321
	Adult	*	60 - 225	10 - 140	34 - 112	119 - 336
2.	6mo	*	61 - 162	34 - 73	43 - 108	135 - 260
	2y	*	61 - 115	35 - 73	40 – 77	147 – 255
	6y	*	65 - 125	37 - 76	39 - 65	165 - 234
	16y	*	104 - 188	54 - 93	46 - 87	178 - 275

Specimen Type:	1,2 Plasma
Reference:	1. Shapira E, Blitzer MG, Miller JB, Africk DK, Eds. Biochemical genetics: a laboratory manual. Oxford, UK: Oxford University Press, 1989:94-5.
	2. Lepage N, McDonald N, Dallaire L, et al. Age-Specific distribution of plasma amino acid concentrations in a healthy pediatric population. Clin Chem 1997; 43: 2397-402
Method(s):	1. Beckman amino-acid analyzer. Beckman 6300 (Beckman Instruments Inc., Palo Alto, CA).
	2. Beckman amino-acid analyzer. Beckman 7300 (Beckman Instruments Inc., Palo Alto, CA).
Comments:	1. Results are mean ± 2SD.
	2. Results are 10 – 90th percentiles in healthy children.
	*See reference for numbers.

AMINO ACIDS (URINE)

Age	n	Male and Female nmol/mg Creatinine			
		Alanine	β-alanine	Anserine	α-amino-adipic acid
Premature (first 6 wk)	*	1320 - 4040	1020 - 3500	- -	70 - 460
0 - 1mo	*	982 - 3055	25 - 288	0 - 3	0 - 180
1 - 24mo	*	767 - 6090	0 - 297	0 - 5	45 - 268
2 - 18y	*	231 - 915	0 - 65	0	2 - 88
Adult	*	240 - 670	0 - 130	0	40 - 110

Specimen Type:	Urine
Reference:	Shapira E, Blitzer MG, Miller JB, Africk DK, Eds. Biochemical genetics: a laboratory manual. Oxford, UK: Oxford University Press, 1989:96-7.
Method(s):	Beckman amino-acid analyzer. Beckman 6300 (Beckman Instruments Inc., Palo Alto, CA).
Comments:	Results are mean ± 2SD. *See reference for numbers.

AMINO ACIDS (URINE)

Age	n	Male and Female nmol/mg Creatinine			
		α-amino-n-butyric acid	γ-amino-butyric acid	β`-amino-isobutyric acid	Arginine
Premature (first 6 wk)	*	50 - 710	20 - 260	50 - 470	190 - 820
0 - 1mo	*	8 - 65	0 - 15	421 - 3133	35 - 214
1 - 24mo	*	30 - 136	0 - 105	802 - 4160	38 - 165
2 - 18y	*	0 - 77	15 - 30	291 - 1482	31 - 109
Adult	*	0 - 90	15 - 30	10 - 510	10 - 90

Specimen Type:	Urine
Reference:	Shapira E, Blitzer MG, Miller JB, Africk DK, Eds. Biochemical genetics: a laboratory manual. Oxford, UK: Oxford University Press, 1989:96-7.
Method(s):	Beckman amino-acid analyzer. Beckman 6300 (Beckman Instruments Inc., Palo Alto, CA).
Comments:	Results are mean ± 2SD. *See reference for numbers.

AMINO ACIDS (URINE)

Age	n	Male and Female nmol/mg Creatinine			
		Asparagine	Aspartic acid	Carnosine	Citrulline
Premature (first 6 wk)	*	1350 - 5250	580 - 1520	260 - 370	240 - 1320
0 - 1mo	*	185 - 1550	336 - 810	97 - 665	27 - 181
1 - 24mo	*	252 - 1280	230 - 685	203 - 635	22 - 180
2 - 18y	*	72 - 332	0 - 120	72 - 402	10 - 99
Adult	*	99 - 470	60 - 240	10 - 90	8 - 50

Specimen Type:	Urine
Reference:	Shapira E, Blitzer MG, Miller JB, Africk DK, Eds. Biochemical genetics: a laboratory manual. Oxford, UK: Oxford University Press, 1989:96-7.
Method(s):	Beckman amino-acid analyzer. Beckman 6300 (Beckman Instruments Inc., Palo Alto, CA).
Comments:	Results are mean ± 2SD. *See reference for numbers.

AMINO ACIDS (URINE)

Age	n	Male and Female nmol/mg Creatinine			
		Cystathionine	Cystine	Ethanolamine	Glutamic Acid
Premature (first 6 wk)	*	260 - 1160	480 - 1690	- -	380 - 3760
0 - 1mo	*	16 - 147	212 - 668	840 - 3400	70 - 1058
1 - 24mo	*	33 - 470	68 - 710	0 - 2230	54 - 590
2 - 18y	*	0 - 26	25 - 125	0 - 530	0 - 176
Adult	*	20 - 50	43 - 210	0 - 520	39 - 330

Specimen Type:	Urine
Reference:	Shapira E, Blitzer MG, Miller JB, Africk DK, Eds. Biochemical genetics: a laboratory manual. Oxford, UK: Oxford University Press, 1989:96-7.
Method(s):	Beckman amino-acid analyzer. Beckman 6300 (Beckman Instruments Inc., Palo Alto, CA).
Comments:	Results are mean ± 2SD. *See reference for numbers.

AMINO ACIDS (URINE)

Age	n	Male and Female nmol/mg Creatinine			
		Glutamine	Glycine	Histidine	Homocystine
Premature (first 6 wk)	*	520 - 1700	7840 - 23600	1240 - 7240	580 - 2230
0 - 1mo	*	393 - 1042	5749 - 16423	908 - 2528	0 - 88
1 - 24mo	*	670 - 1562	3023 - 11148	815 - 7090	6 - 67
2 - 18y	*	369 - 1014	897 - 4500	644 - 2430	0 - 32
Adult	*	190 - 510	730 - 4160	460 - 1430	0 - 32

Specimen Type:	Urine
Reference:	Shapira E, Blitzer MG, Miller JB, Africk DK, Eds. Biochemical genetics: a laboratory manual. Oxford, UK: Oxford University Press, 1989:96-7.
Method(s):	Beckman amino-acid analyzer. Beckman 6300 (Beckman Instruments Inc., Palo Alto, CA).
Comments:	Results are mean ± 2SD.
	*See reference for numbers.

AMINO ACIDS (URINE)

Age	n	Male and Female nmol/mg Creatinine			
		Hydroxylysine	Hydroxyproline	Isoleucine	Leucine
Premature (first 6 wk)	*	--	560 - 5640	250 - 640	190 - 790
0 - 1mo	*	10 - 125	40 - 440	125 - 390	78 - 195
1 - 24mo	*	0 - 97	0 - 4010	38 - 342	70 - 570
2 - 18y	*	40 - 102	0 - 3300	10 - 126	30 - 500
Adult	*	40 - 90	0 - 26	16 - 180	30 - 150

Specimen Type:	Urine
Reference:	Shapira E, Blitzer MG, Miller JB, Africk DK, Eds. Biochemical genetics: a laboratory manual. Oxford, UK: Oxford University Press, 1989:96-7.
Method(s):	Beckman amino-acid analyzer. Beckman 6300 (Beckman Instruments Inc., Palo Alto, CA).
Comments:	Results are mean ± 2SD. *See reference for numbers.

AMINO ACIDS (URINE)

Age	n	Male and Female nmol/mg Creatinine			
		Lysine	Methionine	1-Methyl-histidine	3-Methyl-histidine
Premature (first 6 wk)	*	1860 - 15460	500 - 1230	170 - 880	420 - 1340
0 - 1mo	*	270 - 1850	342 - 880	96 - 499	189 - 680
1 - 24mo	*	189 - 850	174 - 1090	106 - 1275	147 - 391
2 - 18y	*	153 - 634	16 - 114	170 - 1688	182 - 365
Adult	*	145 - 634	38 - 210	170 - 1680	160 - 520

Specimen Type:	Urine
Reference:	Shapira E, Blitzer MG, Miller JB, Africk DK, Eds. Biochemical genetics: a laboratory manual. Oxford, UK: Oxford University Press, 1989:96-7.
Method(s):	Beckman amino-acid analyzer. Beckman 6300 (Beckman Instruments Inc., Palo Alto, CA).
Comments:	Results are mean ± 2SD. *See reference for numbers.

AMINO ACIDS (URINE)

Age	n	Male and Female nmol/mg Creatinine			
		Ornithine	Phenylalanine	Phospho-ethanolamine	Phospho- serine
Premature (first 6 wk)	*	260 - 3350	920 - 2280	80 - 340	500 - 1690
0 - 1mo	*	118 - 554	91 - 457	0 - 155	150 - 339
1 - 24mo	*	55 - 364	175 - 1340	108 - 533	112 - 304
2 - 18y	*	31 -91	61 - 314	18 - 150	70 - 138
Adult	*	20 - 80	51 - 250	20 - 100	40 - 510

Specimen Type:	Urine
Reference:	Shapira E, Blitzer MG, Miller JB, Africk DK, Eds. Biochemical genetics: a laboratory manual. Oxford, UK: Oxford University Press, 1989:96-7.
Method(s):	Beckman amino-acid analyzer. Beckman 6300 (Beckman Instruments Inc., Palo Alto, CA).
Comments:	Results are mean ± 2SD. *See reference for numbers.

AMINO ACIDS (URINE)

Age	n	Male and Female nmol/mg Creatinine			
		Proline	Sarcosine	Serine	Taurine
Premature (first 6 wk)	*	1350 - 10460	0	1680 - 6000	5190 - 23620
0 - 1mo	*	370 - 2323	0 - 56	1444 - 3661	1650 - 6220
1 - 24mo	*	254 - 2195	30 - 358	845 - 3190	545 - 3790
2 - 18y	*	0	0 - 26	362 - 1100	639 - 1866
Adult	*	0	0 - 80	240 - 670	380 - 1850

Specimen Type:	Urine
Reference:	Shapira E, Blitzer MG, Miller JB, Africk DK, Eds. Biochemical genetics: a laboratory manual. Oxford, UK: Oxford University Press, 1989:96-7.
Method(s):	Beckman amino-acid analyzer. Beckman 6300 (Beckman Instruments Inc., Palo Alto, CA).
Comments:	Results are mean ± 2SD. *See reference for numbers.

AMINO ACIDS (URINE)

Age	n	Male and Female nmol/mg Creatinine			
		Threonine	Tryptophan	Tyrosine	Valine
Premature (first 6 wk)	*	840 - 5700	0	1090 - 6780	180 - 890
0 - 1mo	*	445 - 1122	0	220 - 1650	113 - 369
1 - 24mo	*	252 - 1528	0 - 93	333 - 1550	99 - 316
2 - 18y	*	121 - 389	0 - 108	122 - 517	58 - 143
Adult	*	130 - 370	0 - 70	90 - 290	27 - 260

Specimen Type:	Urine
Reference:	Shapira E, Blitzer MG, Miller JB, Africk DK, Eds. Biochemical genetics: a laboratory manual. Oxford, UK: Oxford University Press, 1989:96-7.
Method(s):	Beckman amino-acid analyzer. Beckman 6300 (Beckman Instruments Inc., Palo Alto, CA).
Comments:	Results are mean ± 2SD. *See reference for numbers.

AMMONIA

Test	Age	n	Male and Female
			μmol/L
1.	All ages	*	9 - 33
2.	Newborn	**	< 50
	Child and adult	**	< 35
3.	< 30 d	87	21 - 95
	1 - 12 mo	91	18 - 74
	1 - 14 y	94	17 - 68
	> 14 y	182	22 - 66
	Men	89	21 - 71
	Women	93	19 - 63

Specimen Type:

1, 2 Plasma

3. Whole blood, potassium EDTA as anticoagulant.

Reference:

1. Children's National Medical Center. Unpublished data.

2. Reference values and SI unit information. The Hospital for Sick Children, Toronto, 1993.

3. Diaz J, Tornel PL, Martinez P. Reference intervals for blood ammonia in healthy subjects, determined by microdiffusion. Clin Chem 1995;41:1048. (Letter)

Method(s):

1, 2 Kodak Ektachem 500 & 700 (Johnson & Johnson, Rochester, NY).

3. Ammonia Checker II; Menarini Diagnostics, Florence, Italy.

Comments:

1. Values in premature infants may go as high as 50 μmol/L. Values are 2.5 - 97.5th percentiles.

*Numbers not given.

2. **Numbers not given.

3. Values provided are 5 - 95th percentiles.

AMYLASE

Test	Age	Male and Female	
		n	U/L
1.	1 - 30d	76	0 - 6
	31 - 182d	110	1 - 17
	183 - 365d	54	6 - 44
	1 - 3y	148	8 - 79
	4 - 9y	96	16 - 91
	10 - 18y	142	19 - 76
2.	0 - 0.2y	55	< 30
	0.2 - 0.5y	81	< 50
	0.5 - 1.0y	170	< 80
3.	1- 19 y	470	30 - 100

Specimen Type:	1, 2 Plasma
Reference:	1. Soldin SJ, Hicks JM, Bailey J, et al. Pediatric reference ranges for amylase. Clin Chem 1995;41:S94. (Abstract)
	2. Soldin SJ, Rakotoarisoa FTS. Pediatric reference ranges for amylase and cholesterol on the Kodak Ektachem 500 in the first year of life. Clin Chem 1996;42:S308. (Abstract)
	3. Lockitch G, Halstead AC, Albersheim S, et al. Age and sex specific pediatric reference intervals for biochemistry analytes as measured with the Ektachem 700 analyzer. Clin Chem 1988;34:1622-5.
Method(s):	1. Hitachi 717 using Boehringer-Mannheim reagents (Boehringer-Mannheim Diagnostics, Indianapolis, IN).
	2, 3 Amylopectin. Ektachem 500 and 700 (Johnson & Johnson, Rochester, NY).
Comments:	1. Study used hospitalized patients and a computerized approach to removing outliers. Values are 2.5 - 97.5th percentiles.
	2. Study used hospitalized patients and a computerized approach to removing outliers. Values are 97.5th percentiles.
	3. The study population was healthy children. Non-parametric methods were used to determine the 0.025 and 0.975 fractiles.

ANDROSTENEDIONE

Test	Age	Male			Female		
		n	ng/dL	nmol/L	n	ng/dL	nmol/L
1.	1 - 5mo	9	5 - 45	0.2 - 1.6	5	5 - 35	0.2 - 1.2
	6 - 11mo	8	5 - 30	0.2 - 1.0	6	5 - 25	0.2 - 0.9
	1 - 5y	31	5 - 45	0.2 - 1.6	18	5 - 40	0.2 - 1.4
	6 - 9y	17	5 - 55	0.2 - 1.9	9	5 - 45	0.2 - 1.6
	10 - 11y	7	10 - 30	0.3 - 1.0	11	25 - 80	0.9 - 2.8
	12 - 14y	31	20 - 85	0.7 - 3.0	23	15 - 175	0.5 - 6.1
	15 - 17y	16	35 - 100	1.2 - 3.5	10	55 - 200	1.9 - 7.0
	Adults	*	50 - 250	1.7 - 8.7	*	50 - 250	1.7 - 8.7
2.	0 – 1d	*	15 - 145	0.5 – 5.0	*	15 – 175	0.5 – 6.0
	1 - 7d	*	20 – 110	0.7 – 3.8	*	25 - 95	0.9 – 3.3
	7 - 28d	*	25 – 160	0.9 – 5.5	*	9 - 90	0.3 – 3.0
	1 – 12mo	*	6 - 90	0.2 – 3.0	*	6 – 145	0.2 – 5.0
	1 - <4y	*	6 - 35	0.2 - 1.2	*	6 - 45	0.2 – 1.5
	4 - <10y (P$_1$)	*	25 - 190	0.8 - 3.0	*	3 – 60	0.1 – 2.0
	P$_2$	*	15 – 120	0.5 – 4.0	*	30 – 145	1.0 - 5.0
	P$_3$	*	18 – 145	0.6 – 5.0	*	30 – 200	1.0 – 7.0
	P$_4$	*	15 – 220	0.5 – 7.5	*	18 – 260	0.6 – 9.0
	P$_5$	*	40 - 260	1.3 – 9.0	*	18 - 260	0.6 – 9.0

Specimen Type:	1.	Serum
	2.	Serum/Plasma
Reference:	1.	Nichols Institute. Pediatric Endocrine Testing, 1993:5.
	2.	Soldin SJ, Rifai N, Hicks JM, Eds. Biochemical Basis of Pediatric Disease 3rd Edition. AACC Press, 1998; 233
Method(s):	1.	Extraction, Chromatography, Radioimmunoassay.
	2.	See reference.
Comments:	1.	Results are 2.5 - 97.5th percentiles.
	2.	Numbers not provided. $P_1 - P_5$ refers to pubertal stages. These ranges are for guidance only. *Numbers not provided.

APOLIPOPROTEIN A-1

Test	Age	Male n	Male g/L	Male mg/dL	Female n	Female g/L	Female mg/dL
1.	5y	*	1.04 - 1.67	104 - 167	*	1.08 - 1.60	108 - 160
	10y	*	1.05 - 1.60	105 - 160	*	1.04 - 1.57	104 - 157
	15y	*	1.02 - 1.57	102 - 157	*	1.04 - 1.56	104 - 156
	20y	*	1.04 - 1.65	104 - 165	*	1.08 - 1.65	108 - 165
2.	4 – 5y	*	1.09 - 1.72	109 - 172	*	1.04 - 1.63	104 - 163
	6 – 11y	*	1.11 - 1.77	111 - 177	*	1.10 - 1.66	110 - 166
	12 – 19y	*	0.99 - 1.65	99 - 165	*	1.05 - 1.80	105 - 180

	Age	Male and Female n	Male and Female g/L	Male and Female mg/dL
3.	2 - 12mo	100	0.79 - 1.87	79 - 187
	2 - 10y	120	1.07 - 1.79	107 - 179

Specimen Type:	1. Plasma 2. Serum 3. Serum
Reference:	1. Kottke BA, Moll PP, Michels VV, et al. Levels of lipids, lipoproteins, and apolipoproteins in a defined population. Mayo Clin Proc 1991;66:1198-1208. 2. Bachorik PS, Lovejoy KL, Carroll MD, et al. Apolipoprotein B and A1 distributions in the United States, 1988-1991: results of the National Health and Nutrition Examination Surevey III (NHANES III). Clin Chem 1997; 43:2364-78 3. Baroni S, Scribano D, Valentini P, et al. Serum apolipoprotein A1, B, CII, CIII, E, and lipoprotein (a) levels in children. Clin Biochem 1996;29:603-5.
Method(s):	1. Radioimmunoassay. See reference. 2. Radial immunodiffusion and rate immunonephelometry. See reference above 3. Behring Nephelometry using Behring reagents (Behring Diagnostics, Westwood, MA)
Comments:	1. Results are 5 - 95th percentiles read off graphs in above reference. *See reference for numbers. 2. Healthy children were studied. The results are the 5 – 95th percentiles. The numbers studied are not provided. 3. Results are the 2.5 - 97.5th percentiles for healthy children.

APOLIPOPROTEIN (a)

Test			Male and Female
1.	Age	n	U/L
	2d	29	0 - 59
	3d	151	0 - 57
	4d	459	0 - 69
	5d	341	0 - 66
	6d	30	0 - 78
	7d	22	0 - 71
2.	Age	n	mg/L
	2 - 12mo	100	0 - 114
	2 - 10y	120	0 - 178

Specimen Type:	1.	Dried blood spot
	2.	Serum
Reference:	1.	Wang XL, Wilcken DEL, Dudman NPB. Neonatal apo A-1, apo-B and apo(a) levels in dried blood spots in an Australian population. Ped Res 1990;28:496-501.
	2.	Baroni S, Scribano D, Valentini P, et al. Serum apolipoprotein A1, B, CII, CIII, E and lipoprotein (a) levels in children. Clin Biochem 1996;29:603-5.
Method(s):	1.	Modification of RIA serum assay for apo(a). (Pharmacia Diagnostics AB, Uppsala, Sweden).
	2.	EIA, Macra Lpa test kit (Strategic Diagnostics, Newark, DE)
Comments:	1.	Healthy neonates were studied. Results are mean ± 2SD.
	2.	Results are the 2.5 - 97.5th percentiles for healthy children.

APOLIPOPROTEIN B

Test	Age	n	Male g/L	Male mg/dL	n	Female g/L	Female mg/dL
1.	5y	*	0.51 - 0.80	51 - 80	*	0.54 - 0.87	54 - 87
	10y	*	0.50 - 0.88	50 - 88	*	0.54 - 0.87	54 - 87
	15y	*	0.48 - 0.85	48 - 85	*	0.54 - 0.87	54 - 87
	20y	*	0.48 - 0.90	48 - 90	*	0.54 - 0.85	54 - 85
2.	4 – 5y	*	0.58 - 1.03	58 - 103	*	0.58 - 1.04	58 - 104
	6 – 11y	*	0.56 - 1.05	56 - 105	*	0.57 - 1.13	57 - 113
	12 – 19y	*	0.55 - 1.10	55 - 110	*	0.53 - 1.19	53 - 119

3.	Age	n	Male and Female mg/dL	Male and Female g/L
	2 - 12mo	100	41 - 105	0.41 - 1.05
	2 - 10y	120	44 - 112	0.44 - 1.12

Specimen Type:
1. Plasma
2. Serum
3. Serum

Reference:
1. Kottke BA, Moll PP, Michels V, et al. Levels of lipids, lipoproteins, and apolipoproteins in a defined population. Mayo Clin Proc 1991;66:1198-1208.

2. Bachorik PS, Lovejoy KL, Carroll MD, et al. Apolipoprotein B and A1 distributions in the United States, 1988-1991: results of the National Health and Nutrition Examination Surevey III (NHANES III). Clin Chem 1997; 43:2364-78

3. Baroni S, Scribano D, Valentini P, et al. Serum apolipoprotein A1, B, CII, CIII, E and lipoprotein (a) levels in children. Clin Biochem 1996;29:603-5.

Method(s):
1. Enzyme linked immunosorbent assay. See reference.

2. Radial immunodiffusion and rate nephelometry. See reference above

3. Behring Nephelometer using Behring reagents (Behring Diagnostics, Westwood, MA)

Comments:
1. Results are 5 - 95th percentiles read off graphs in above reference. *See reference for numbers.

2. Healthy children were studied. The results are the 5 – 95th percentiles. The numbers studied are not provided.

3. Results are the 2.5th and 97.5th percentiles for healthy children.

APOLIPOPROTEIN CII

Age	Male and Female	
	n	mg/L
2 - 12mo	100	15 - 79
2 - 10y	120	9 - 73

Specimen Type:	Serum
Reference:	Baroni S, Scribano D, Valentini P, et al. Serum apolipoprotein A1, B, CII, CIII, E, and lipoprotein (a) levels in children. Clin Biochem 1996;29:603-5.
Method(s):	Turbidimetric immunoassay (Turbilinear "Eiken" Poli, Milan, Italy)
Comments:	Results are the 2.5 - 97.5th percentiles for healthy children.

APOLIPOPROTEIN CIII

	Male and Female	
Age	n	mg/L
2 - 12mo	100	18 - 134
2 - 10y	120	25 – 113

Specimen Type:	Serum
Reference:	Baroni S, Scribano D, Valentini P, et al. Serum apolipoprotein A1, B, CII, CIII, E, and lipoprotein (a) levels in children. Clin Biochem 1996;29:603-5.
Method(s):	Turbidimetric immunoassay (Turbilinear "Eiken" Poli, Milan, Italy)
Comments:	Results are the 2.5 - 97.5th percentiles for healthy children.

APOLIPOPROTEIN E

	Male and Female		
Age	n	mg/L
2 - 12mo	100	23 - 59
2 - 10y	120	19 - 59

Specimen Type:	Serum
Reference:	Baroni S, Scribano D, Valentini P, et al. Serum apolipoprotein A1, B, CII, CIII, E, and lipoprotein (a) levels in children. Clin Biochem 1996;29:603-5.
Method(s):	Turbidimetric immunoassay (Turbilinear "Eiken" Poli, Milan, Italy)
Comments:	Results are the 2.5 - 97.5th percentiles for healthy children.

ASPARTATE AMINOTRANSFERASE
(AST, SGOT)

Test	Age	Male		Female	
		n	U/L	n	U/L
1.	1 - 7d	69	30 - 100	52	24 - 95
	8 - 30d	148	20 - 70	84	24 - 72
	1 - 3mo	160	22 - 63	131	20 - 64
	4 - 6mo	133	13 - 65	83	20 - 63
	7 - 12mo	131	25 - 55	142	22 - 63
2.	1 - 3y	50*	20 - 60	50*	20 - 60
	5 - 6y	40*	15 - 50	40*	15 - 50
	7 - 9y	80*	15 - 40	80*	15 - 40
	10 - 11y	27	10 - 60	34	10 - 40
	12 - 13y	31	15 - 40	49	10 - 30
	14 - 15y	26	15 - 40	52	10 - 30
	16 - 19y	40	15 - 45	61	5 - 30
3.	1 - 30d	74	< 51	57	< 49
	31 - 365d	83	< 65	71	< 79
	1 - 3y	134	< 56	108	< 69
	4 - 6y	85	< 48	84	< 59
	7 - 9y	122	< 42	96	< 41
	10 - 12y	104	< 38	62	< 37
	13 - 15y	88	< 39	86	< 32
	16 - 18y	62	< 39	78	< 30

Specimen Type:	1, 3	Plasma or serum
	2	Plasma
Reference:	1.	Soldin SJ, Savwoir TV, Guo Y. Pediatric reference ranges for alkaline phosphatase, aspartate aminotransferase, and alanine aminotransferase in children less than 1 year old on the Vitros 500. Clin Chem 1997;43:S199. (Abstract)
	2.	Lockitch G, Halstead AC, Albersheim S, et al. Age and sex specific pediatric reference intervals for biochemistry analytes as measured with the Ektachem 700 analyzer. Clin Chem 1988;34:1622-5.
	3.	Soldin SJ, Hicks JM, Bailey J, et al. Pediatric reference ranges for AST. Clin Chem 1995;44:S94. (Abstract)
Method(s):	1, 2	Ektachem 500 (1) and 700 (2) (Johnson & Johnson, Rochester, NY).
	3.	Measured on the Hitachi 747 using Boehringer-Mannheim reagents (Boehringer-Mannheim Diagnostics, Indianapolis, IN).
Comments:	1, 3	Study used hospitalized patients and a computerized approach adapted from the Hoffmann technique to obtain the 2.5 - 97.5th percentiles (Test 1) and 97.5th percentile (Test 3).
	2.	The study population was healthy children. Non-parametric methods were used to determine the 0.025 and 0.975 fractiles.

*No significant differences were found for males and females.
These ranges were therefore derived from combined data.

BASE EXCESS		
		Male and Female
Age	**n**	**mmol/L**
Newborn	*	-10 to -2
Infant	*	-7 to -1
Child	*	-4 to +2
Thereafter	*	-3 to +3

Specimen Type:	Whole blood
Reference:	Behrman RE, Ed. Nelson textbook of pediatrics, 14th ed. Philadelphia, PA: W.B. Saunders Company, 1992:1803.
Method(s):	Not described.
Comments:	*Numbers not given.

BILE ACIDS (TOTAL)
(TOTAL 3-α-HYDROXY BILE ACIDS)

		Male and Female
Age	n	μmol/L
1	42	11 - 69
3	35	1 - 41
6	50	1 - 30
9	36	1 - 28
12	37	1 - 37
Adult	7	1 - 7

Specimen Type:	Serum
Reference:	McGraw C, Ellinor YM, Heubi JE. Reference ranges for total serum bile acids in infants. Clin Chem 1996;42:S307 (Abstract).
Method(s):	Nonradioactive enzymatic spectrophotometric method. "Enzabile," adapted for use on the Hitachi 705 analyzer. (Boehringer-Mannheim Diagnostics, Indianapolis, IN)
Comments:	Results are 2.5 - 97.5th percentiles. Population studied was a nonfasting, healthy population.

BILIRUBIN
(CONJUGATED)

Test	Age	Male and Female		
		n	μmol/L	mg/dL
1.	Neonates	*	< 10	< 0.6
	> Neonate	*	< 2	< 0.1
2.	Preterm infants (1-6 d)	30	< 10	< 0.6

Specimen Type:	1,2	Serum
Reference:	1.	Reference values and SI information. The Hospital for Sick Children, Toronto, Canada, 1993:359.
	2.	Lockitch G, Halstead AC, Albersheim S, et al. Age and sex specific pediatric reference intervals for biochemistry analytes as measured with the Ektachem 700 analyzer. Clin Chem 1988;34:1622-5.
Method(s):	1,2	Kodak Ektachem 700 (Johnson & Johnson, Rochester, NY).
Comments:	1.	*Numbers not given.
	2.	Results are 97.5th percentile.

BILIRUBIN
(TOTAL)

		Male and Female		
Test	**Age**	**n**	**μmol/L**	**mg/dL**
1.	Birth - 1d	*	< 100	< 5.8
	1 - 2d	*	< 140	< 8.2
	3 - 5d	*	< 200	< 11.7
	1mo - adult	*	< 17	< 1.0
2.	Bottle fed infants	2416**	< 212	< 12.4
	Breast fed infants	2416**	< 253	< 14.8

Specimen Type:	1,2 Serum
Reference:	1. Reference values and SI information. The Hospital for Sick Children, Toronto, Canada, 1993:359.
	2. Maisels MJ, Gifford K. Normal serum bilirubin levels in the newborn and the effect of breast-feeding. Pediatrics 1986;78:837-43.
Method(s):	1. Kodak Ektachem 700 (Johnson & Johnson, Rochester, NY).
	2. Modified diazo method on ACA III (DuPont Co., Clinical Systems Division, Wilmington, DE).
Comments:	1. Should decrease to adult values by day 10 (breast-fed infants may take longer). Values in premature infants may be higher than in term infants and may reach peak concentrations at later times. *Numbers not provided.
	2. **2,416 consecutive infants admitted to the well-baby nursery studied. This number includes both formula- and breast-fed infants. Results are 97th percentile. Breast feeding was significantly associated with hyperbilirubinemia.

C1 ESTERASE INHIBITOR

Test	Age	Males		Females	
		n	mg/L	n	mg/L
1.	0 – 30d	27	75 – 170	19	80 - 150
	31 – 182d	39	105 – 279	49	105 - 229
	6mo - <4y	106	145 - 268	103	159 - 280
	4 - <7y	75	140 - 252	48	120 – 269
	7 - <10y	54	135 - 270	31	136 – 190
	10 - <13y	60	118 – 209	61	142 – 211
	13 - <16y	68	130 – 229	56	127 – 201
	16 – 18y	35	130 – 216	47	140 - 200

Specimen Type:	1.	Serum/Plasma
Reference:	1.	Soldin SJ, Hicks JM, Bailey J, et al. Pediatric reference ranges for Estradiol and C1 Esterase Inhibitor. Clin Chem 1998;44:A17. (Abstract)
Method(s):	1,	Diasorin kit. (Diasorin Corp., Stillwater, MN.)
Comments:	1.	The Study used serum/plasma from hospitalized patients and employed Chauvenet's criteria for removing outliers and a computerized approach adapted from the Hoffmann technic to obtain the 2.5 – 97.5[th] percentiles.

CALCIUM

Test	Age	Male			Female		
		n	mg/dL	mmol/L	n	mg/dL	mmol/L
1.	0 - 7d	293	7.3 – 11.4	1.83 - 2.85	259	7.5 – 11.3	1.88 - 2.83
	8 – 30d	434	8.6 – 11.7	2.15 - 2.93	264	8.4 – 11.9	2.10 - 2.98
	31 – 90d	371	8.5 – 11.3	2.13 - 2.83	265	8.0 – 11.1	2.00 - 2.78
	91 – 180d	186	8.3 – 11.4	2.08 - 2.85	222	7.7 – 11.5	1.93 - 2.88
	181 – 365d	429	7.7 – 11.0	1.93 - 2.75	362	7.8 – 11.1	1.95 - 2.78
2.	0 - 5d (< 2.5 kg)	50*	7.9 - 10.7	1.96 - 2.66	50*	7.9 - 10.7	1.96 - 2.66
	1 - 3y	50*	8.7 - 9.8	2.17 - 2.44	50*	8.7 - 9.8	2.17 - 2.44
	4 - 6y	38*	8.8 - 10.1	2.19 - 2.51	38*	8.8 - 10.1	2.19 - 2.51
	7 - 9y	72*	8.8 - 10.1	2.19 - 2.51	72*	8.8 - 10.1	2.19 - 2.51
	10 - 11y	62*	8.9 - 10.1	2.22 - 2.51	62*	8.9 - 10.1	2.22 - 2.51
	12 - 13y	73*	8.8 - 10.6	2.19 - 2.64	73*	8.8 - 10.6	2.19 - 2.64
	14 - 15y	91*	9.2 - 10.7	2.29 - 2.66	91*	9.2 - 10.7	2.29 - 2.66
	16 - 19y	107*	8.9 - 10.7	2.22 - 2.66	107*	8.9 - 10.7	2.22 - 2.66
3.	1 - 30d	62	8.5 - 10.6	2.12 - 2.64	66	8.4 - 10.6	2.10 - 2.64
	31 - 365d	83	8.7 - 10.5	2.17 - 2.62	66	8.9 - 10.5	2.22 - 2.62
	1 - 3y	126	8.8 - 10.6	2.19 - 2.64	119	8.5 - 10.4	2.12 - 2.59
	4 - 6y	112	8.8 - 10.6	2.19 - 2.64	106	8.5 - 10.6	2.12 - 2.64
	7 - 9y	117	8.7 - 10.3	2.17 - 2.57	107	8.5 - 10.3	2.12 - 2.57
	10 - 12y	135	8.7 - 10.2	2.17 - 2.54	115	8.6 - 10.2	2.15 - 2.64
	13 - 15y	109	8.5 - 10.2	2.12 - 2.54	110	8.4 - 10.0	2.10 - 2.50
	16 - 18y	95	8.4 - 10.3	2.10 - 2.57	122	8.6 - 9.8	2.15 - 2.45

Specimen Type:	1,3. Plasma/Serum 2. Serum
Reference:	1. Soldin SJ, Morse AS. Pediatric Reference Ranges for Calcium and Triglycerides in Children <1 Year Old Using the Vitros 500 Analyzer. Clin Chem 1998;44:A16. (Abstract) 2. Lockitch G, Halstead AC, Albersheim S, et al. Age and sex specific pediatric reference intervals for biochemistry analytes as measured with the Ektachem 700 analyzer. Clin Chem 1988;34:1622-5. 3. Soldin SJ, Hicks JM, Bailey J, et al. Pediatric reference ranges for calcium on the Hitachi 747 Analyzer. Clin Chem 1997;43:S198. (Abstract)
Method(s):	1, 2. Arsenazo III dye method. Ektachem 700 (Johnson & Johnson, Rochester, NY). 3. Cresolphthalein complexone. Hitachi 747 Boehringer-Mannheim reagents (Boehringer-Mannheim Diagnostics, Indianapolis, IN).
Comments:	1, 3. Study used hospitalized patients and a computerized approach to removing outliers. Values are 2.5 - 97.5th percentiles. 2. From normal healthy children. Values are 2.5 - 97.5th percentiles. *No significant differences were found for males and females. These ranges were therefore derived from combined data.

CALCIUM, IONIZED

Test	Age	n	Male mg/dL	Male mmol/L	Female mg/dL	Female mmol/L
1.	0 - 1mo	207	3.9 - 6.0	1.0 - 1.5	3.9 - 6.0	1.0 - 1.5
	1 - 6mo	96	3.7 - 5.9	0.95 - 1.5	3.7 - 5.9	0.95 - 1.5
2.	1 - 19y	*	4.9 - 5.5	1.22 - 1.37		
	20y – adult	*	4.75 - 5.3	1.18 - 1.32		
	1 - 17y	*			4.9 - 5.5	1.22 - 1.37
	18y – adult	*			4.75 - 5.3	1.18 - 1.32

Specimen Type:	1,2 Whole blood
Reference:	1. Snell J, Greeley C, Colaco A, et al. Pediatric reference ranges for arterial pH, whole blood electrolytes and glucose. Clin Chem 1993:39;1173. (Abstract) 2. Burritt MF, Slockbower JM, Forsman RW, et al. Pediatric reference intervals for 19 biologic variables in healthy children. Mayo Clinic Proceedings 1990:65;329-36.
Method(s):	1. Ciba Corning 288 Blood Gas System. (Ciba Corning Diagnostics, East Walpole, MA.) 2. Ion selective electrode Radiometer ICA 1. (Radiometer America, Inc., Cleveland, OH.)
Comments:	1. Study used hospitalized patients and a computerized approach to removing outliers. Values are 2.5 - 97.5th percentiles. 2. From normal healthy children. Values are 2.5 - 97.5th percentiles. *See manuscript for numbers.

CARBON DIOXIDE (CO₂)

Test	Age	Male and Female mmol/L
1.	0 - 1wk	17 – 26
	1wk - 1mo	17 – 27
	1 - 6mo	17 – 29
	6mo - 1y	18 – 29
	1y	20 – 31
2.	Infants	13 – 29
	Adults	24 – 30

Specimen Type:	1. Plasma 2. Cord blood
Reference:	1. Greeley C, Snell J, Colaco A, et al. Pediatric reference ranges for electrolytes and creatinine. Clin Chem 1993;39:1172. (Abstract) 2. Perkins SL, Livesey JF, Belcher J. Reference intervals for 21 clinical chemistry analytes in arterial and venous umbilical cord blood. Clin Chem 1993;39:1041-4.
Method(s):	1. Kodak Ektachem 700 (Johnson & Johnson, Rochester, NY). 2. Hitachi 737, Boehringer-Mannheim reagents (Boehringer-Mannheim, Montreal, Canada).
Comments:	1. Study used hospitalized patients and a computerized approach to removing outliers. N ≥ 100 in all of the above. Values are 2.5 - 97.5th percentiles. 2. Study used 397 infants (209 girls and 188 boys delivered between 37 and 41 weeks gestation). Results are 2.5 - 97.5th percentiles.

CARBON DIOXIDE, PARTIAL PRESSURE
(pCO$_2$)

		Male and Female	
Age	n	mmHg	kPa
Newborn	*	27 - 40	3.6 - 5.3
Infant	*	27 - 41	3.6 - 5.5
Thereafter	*	32 - 48	4.3 - 6.4

Specimen Type:	Whole blood
Reference:	Behrman RE, Ed. Nelson textbook of pediatrics, 14th ed. Philadelphia, PA: WB Saunders Company, 1992:1804.
Method(s):	Not given.
Comments:	*Numbers not provided.

CARNITINE
(TOTAL)

Test	Age	Male		Female	
		n	µmol/L	n	µmol/L
1.	1 - 7d	*	17 - 46	*	17 - 46
	2y	*	24 - 66	*	24 - 66
	> 2y	*	37 - 89	*	30 - 73
2.	1 - 12mo	12	15 - 39	12	15 - 39
	1 - 7y	27	18 - 37	27	18 - 37
	7 - 15y	9	31 - 43	9	31 - 43

Specimen Type:	1.	Serum
	2.	Plasma
Reference:	1.	Mayo Medical Laboratories test catalogue, 1994:78.
	2.	Bonnefont JP, Specola NP, Vassault A, et al. The fasting test in pediatrics: application to the diagnosis of pathological hypo- and hyperketotic states. Eur J Pediatr 1990;150:80-5.
Method(s):	1.	Radioisotope enzymatic.
	2.	Radioisotopic assay. See reference
Comments:		*Note:* Free carnitine normally comprises 60 - 80% of the total carnitine.
	1.	The total carnitine minus the free carnitine gives the esterified carnitine.
		*Numbers not provided.
	2.	The above results are 10 - 90th percentiles and refer to 15h fasting values. For 20 and 24h fasting values, see reference.

CERULOPLASMIN

Test	Age	Male		Female	
		n	mg/L	n	mg/L
1.	0 - 5d	73*	50 - 260	73*	50 - 260
	1 - 3y	51*	240 - 460	51*	240 - 460
	4 - 6y	39*	240 - 420	39*	240 - 420
	7 - 9y	39*	240 - 400	39*	240 - 400
	10 - 13y	36	220 - 360	45	230 - 430
	14 - 19y	46	140 - 340	66	200 - 450
2.	1 - 30d	35	70 - 230	36	30 - 250
	31 - 365d	119	140 - 440	87	140 - 390
	1 - 3 y	127	230 - 510	114	260 - 490
	4 - 6y	99	260 - 510	81	240 - 490
	7 - 9y	75	230 - 470	84	210 - 440
	10 - 12y	69	190 - 460	90	190 - 440
	13 - 15y	73	180 - 450	72	190 - 420
	16 - 18y	49	180 - 410	73	200 - 450

Specimen Type:
1. Serum
2. Serum, Plasma

Reference:
1. Lockitch G, Halstead AC, Quigley G, et al. Age and sex specific pediatric reference intervals: study design and methods illustrated by measurement of serum proteins with the Behring LN Nephelometer. Clin Chem 1988;34:1618-21.

2. Soldin SJ, Hicks JM, Bailey J, et al. Pediatric reference ranges for β2-microglobulin and ceruloplasmin. Clin Chem 1997;43:S199. (Abstract)

Method(s):
1. Nephelometry using Behring antisera and Behring LN Nephelometer (Behring Diagnostics, Hoechst Canada, Inc., Montreal, Canada).

2. Behring Nephelometer with Behring reagents (Behring Diagnostics, Westwood MA)

Comments:
1. Healthy normal children. Results represent the 0.025 - 0.975 fractiles. Males and females had similar ranges from 0 - 9y and numbers quoted are combined for these age ranges.

   *No significant differences were found for males and females. These ranges were therefore derived from combined data.

2. Study used hospitalized patients and a computerized approach adapted from the Hoffmann technique. Values are the 2.5 - 97.5th percentiles.

CHLORIDE

Test	Age	n	Male and Female mmol/L
1.	0 - 1wk	≥ 100	96 - 111
	1wk - 1mo	≥ 100	96 - 110
	1 - 6mo	≥ 100	96 - 110
	6mo - 1y	≥ 100	96 - 108
	over 1y	≥ 100	96 - 109
2.	1 - 17y	*	102 - 112
	18 - Adult	*	100 - 108

Specimen Type:	1. Plasma 2. Serum
Reference:	1. Greeley C, Snell J, Colaco A, et al. Pediatric reference ranges for electrolytes and creatinine. Clin Chem 1993;39:1172. (Abstract) 2. Burritt MF, Slockbower JM, Forsman BS, et al. Pediatric reference intervals for 19 biologic variables in healthy children. Mayo Clinic Proceedings 1990;65:329-36.
Method(s):	1. Kodak Ektachem (Johnson & Johnson, Rochester, NY). 2. Coulometric-Beckman Astra 8 (Beckman Instruments, Inc., Palo Alto, CA).
Comments:	1. Study used hospitalized patients and a computerized approach to removing outliers. Values are 2.5 - 97.5th percentiles. N ≥ 100 in all of the above. 2. From normal children healthy children. Values are 2.5 - 97.5th percentiles. *See reference for numbers.

CHOLESTEROL

Test	Age	Male			Female		
		n	mg/dL	mmol/L	n	mg/dL	mmol/L
1.	0 - 1mo	37	45 - 177	1.16 - 4.58	27	63 - 198	1.63 - 5.12
	2 - 6mo	354	60 - 197	1.55 - 5.09	243	66 - 218	1.71 - 5.64
	7 - 12mo	401	89 - 208	2.30 - 5.39	252	74 - 218	1.91 - 5.64
2.	1 - 3y	49*	44 - 181	1.15 - 4.70	49*	44 - 181	1.15 - 4.70
	4 - 6y	38*	108 - 187	2.80 - 4.80	38*	108 - 187	2.80 - 4.80
	7 - 9y	72*	112 - 247	2.90 - 6.40	72*	112 - 247	2.90 - 6.40
	10 - 11y	28	125 - 230	3.25 - 5.95	34	127 - 244	3.30 - 6.30
	12 - 13y	32	127 - 230	3.30 - 5.95	40	125 - 213	3.25 - 5.55
	14 - 15y	39	106 - 224	2.75 - 5.80	50	130 - 213	3.35 - 5.55
	16 - 19y	41	110 - 220	2.85 - 5.70	68	106 - 217	2.75 - 5.60
3.	1 - 30d	62	54 - 151	1.40 - 3.90	74	62 - 155	1.60 - 4.01
	31 - 182d	77	81 - 147	2.09 - 3.80	75	62 - 141	1.60 - 3.65
	183 - 365d	53	76 - 179	1.97 - 4.63	45	76 - 216	1.97 - 5.59
	1 - 3y	136	85 - 182	2.20 - 4.71	111	108 - 193	2.79 - 4.99
	4 - 6y	112	110 - 217	2.84 - 5.61	113	106 - 193	2.74 - 4.99
	7 - 9y	124	110 - 211	2.84 - 5.46	104	104 - 210	2.69 - 5.43
	10 - 12y	111	105 - 223	2.72 - 5.77	109	105 - 218	2.72 - 5.64
	13 - 15y	126	91 - 204	2.35 - 5.28	105	108 - 205	2.79 - 5.30
	16 - 18y	112	82 - 192	2.12 - 4.97	110	92 - 234	2.38 - 6.05

Specimen Type:	1-3	Plasma or Serum
Reference:	1.	Soldin SJ, Rakotoarisoa FTS. Pediatric reference ranges for amylase and cholesterol on the Kodak Ektachem 500 in the first year of life. Clin Chem 1996;42:S308. (Abstract)
	2.	Lockitch G, Halstead AC, Albersheim S, et al. Age and sex specific pediatric reference intervals for biochemistry analytes as measured with the Ektachem 700 analyzer. Clin Chem 1988;34:1622-5.
	3.	Hicks JM, Bailey J, Beatey J, et al. Pediatric reference ranges for cholesterol. Clin Chem 1996;42:S307. (Abstract)
Method(s):	1, 2	Cholesterol oxidase method. Ektachem 700 (Johnson & Johnson, Rochester, NY).
	3.	Boehringer-Mannheim reagents on the Hitachi 747 analyzer. (Boehringer-Mannheim Diagnostics, Indianapolis, IN.)
Comments:	1, 3	Values are 2.5 - 97.5th percentiles. Study used hospitalized patients and a computerized appoach to removing outliers.
	2.	The study population was healthy children. Non-parametric methods were used to determine the reference values. The central 95% were used. *Males and females were not studied separately; n refers to the total number of males *and* females studied in each age group.

COMPLEMENT FRACTION
(C_{1r})

Test	Age	Male and Female	
		n	mg/L
1.	Terun newborn cord blood	125	27 - 65
	>18y	31	25 - 140

Specimen Type:	1	Plasma (EDTA or citrate)
Reference:	1.	Sonntag J, Brandenburg U, Polzehl D, et al. Complement System in Healthy Term Newborns: Reference Values in Umbilical Cord Blood. Ped Develop Path 1998;1:131-5
Method(s):	1.	Single radial immunodiffusion (Binding Site, Birmingham, UK)
Comments:	1.	Studies were performed on cord blood obtained from 125 healthy term newborns. Results are 5-95th percentiles.

COMPLEMENT FRACTION
(C₂)

Test	Age	Male and Female	
		n	mg/L
1.	Terun newborn cord blood	125	12 - 24
	>18y	31	18 - 40

Specimen Type:	1	Plasma (EDTA or citrate)
Reference:	1.	Sonntag J, Brandenburg U, Polzehl D, et al. Complement System in Healthy Term Newborns: Reference Values in Umbilical Cord Blood. Ped Develop Path 1998;1:131-5
Method(s):	1.	Single radial immunodiffusion (Binding Site, Birmingham, UK)
Comments:	1.	Studies were performed on cord blood obtained from 125 healthy term newborns. Results are 5-95th percentiles.

COMPLEMENT FRACTION
(C_{3a})

Test	Age	Male and Female	
		n	µg/L
1.	Term newborn cord blood	125	4 - 255
	>18y	31	0 - 161

Specimen Type:	1	Plasma (EDTA or citrate)
Reference:	1.	Sonntag J, Brandenburg U, Polzehl D, et al. Complement System in Healthy Term Newborns: Reference Values in Umbilical Cord Blood. Ped Develop Path 1998;1:131-5
Method(s):	1.	Enzyme immunoassay (EIA: Fa. Progen Biotechnik GmbH, Heidelberg, Germany).
Comments:	1.	Studies were performed on cord blood obtained from 125 healthy term newborns. Results are 5-95th percentiles.

COMPLEMENT FRACTION
(C_{3c})

Test	Age	Male		Female	
		n	g/L	n	g/L
1.	0 – 6mo	70	0.37 – 1.00	71	0.37 – 0.90
	6mo – 3y	121	0.57 – 1.19	117	0.48 – 1.09
	4 – 6y	66	0.67 – 1.27	54	0.64 – 1.22
	7 – 9y	70	0.77 – 1.40	38	0.69 – 1.24
	10 – 12y	82	0.74 – 1.07	73	0.73 – 1.27
	13 – 15y	68	0.65 – 1.34	74	0.74 – 1.18
	16 – 18y	36	0.76 – 1.25	57	0.61 – 1.20

Test	Age	Male and Female	
		n	g/L
2.	Healthy infants	32	0.30 - 0.98
3.	0 - 5d	73	0.26 - 1.04
	1 - 19y	334	0.51 - 0.95
	Adult	30	0.45 - 0.83

Specimen Type:	1,2. Serum 3. Serum/Plasma
Reference:	1. Soldin SJ, Hicks JM, Bailey J, et al. Pediatric Reference Ranges for Complement Factors C3c and C4. Clin Chem 1998;44:A14. (Abstract) 2. Zilow G, Zilow EP, Burger R, et al. Complement activation in newborn infants with early onset infection. Ped Res 1993;34:199-203. 3. Lockitch G, Halstead AC, Quigley G, et al. Age and sex specific pediatric reference intervals: study design and methods illustrated by measurement of serum proteins with the Behring LN Nephelometer. Clin Chem 1988;34:1618-21.
Method(s):	1. Behring nephelometer using Behring kits (Behring Diagnostics Inc. Westwood, MA) 2. Radial Immunodiffusion (Behring Diagnostics, Frankfurt, Germany). 3. Nephelometric on Behring LN Nephelometer (Behring Diagnostics, Hoechst Canada, Inc., Montreal).
Comments:	1. The study used serum/plasma from hospitalized patients and employed Chauvenet's criteria for removing outliers and a computerized approach adapted from the Hoffmann technic to obtain the $2.5 - 97.5^{th}$ percentiles. 2. C_3 reported in serum from normal neonates. Results are 0 - 100th percentiles. 3. Healthy children and adults. Results are 0.025 - 0.975 fractiles

COMPLEMENT FRACTION
(C$_4$)

Test	Age	Male and Female	
		n	**g/L**
1.	0 - 5d	73	0.06 - 0.37
	1 - 19y	334	0.08 - 0.44
	Adult	30	0.11 - 0.41

Test	Age	Male		Female	
		n	**g/L**	**n**	**g/L**
2.	0 – 6mo	68	0.10 – 0.31	71	0.11 – 0.28
	6mo – 3y	121	0.15 – 0.53	116	0.15 – 0.47
	4 – 6y	66	0.22 – 0.52	54	0.19 – 0.46
	7 – 9y	69	0.19 – 0.39	38	0.18 – 0.46
	10 – 12y	82	0.20 – 0.40	73	0.16 – 0.52
	13 – 15y	68	0.19 – 0.57	74	0.18 – 0.41
	16 – 18y	36	0.19 – 0.42	57	0.12 – 0.44

Specimen Type:
1. Serum
2. Serum/Plasma

Reference:
1. Lockitch G, Halstead AC, Quigley G, et al. Age and sex specific pediatric reference intervals: study design and methods illustrated by measurement of serum proteins with the Behring LN Nephelometer. Clin Chem 1988;34:1618-21.
2. Soldin SJ, Hicks JM, Bailey J, et al. Pediatric Reference Ranges for Complement Factors C3c and C4. Clin Chem 1998;44:A14. (Abstract)

Method(s):
1,2. Nephelometric, Behring LN Nephelometer (Behring Diagnostics, Hoechst Canada, Inc., Montreal, and Westwood, MA)

Comments:
1. Normal healthy children. Values provided are 0.025 - 0.975 fractiles.
2. The study used serum/plasma from hospitalized patients and employed Chauvenet's criteria for removing outliers and a computerized approach adapted from the Hoffmann technic to obtain the 2.5 – 97.5[th] percentiles.

COMPLEMENT FRACTION
(C$_5$)

| Test | Age | Male and Female | |
		n	mg/L
1.	Term newborn cord blood	125	64 - 127
	>18y	31	83 - 169

Specimen Type:	1	Plasma (EDTA or citrate)
Reference:	1.	Sonntag J, Brandenburg U, Polzehl D, et al. Complement System in Healthy Term Newborns: Reference Values in Umbilical Cord Blood. Ped and Develop Path 1998;1:131-5
Method(s):	1.	Single radial immunodiffusion (Binding Site, Birmingham, UK)
Comments:	1.	Studies were performed on cord blood obtained from 125 healthy term newborns. Results are 5-95th percentiles.

COMPLEMENT FRACTION
(C_{5a})

Test	Age	Male and Female	
		n	µg/L
1.	Term newborn cord blood	125	0.11 – 1.19
	>18y	31	0.00 – 0.62

Specimen Type:	1	Plasma (EDTA or citrate)
Reference:	1.	Sonntag J, Brandenburg U, Polzehl D, et al. Complement System in Healthy Term Newborns: Reference Values in Umbilical Cord Blood. Ped and Develop Path 1998;1:131-5
Method(s):	1.	Specific Sandwich EIA (FA. Behring, Marburg, Germany)
Comments:	1.	Studies were performed on cord blood obtained from 125 healthy term newborns. Results are 5-95th percentiles.

COMPLEMENT FRACTION (C_7)			
		Male and Female	
Test	**Age**	**n**	**mg/L**
1.	Term newborn cord blood	125	32 - 89
	>18y	31	35 - 79

Specimen Type:	1	Plasma (EDTA or citrate)
Reference:	1.	Sonntag J, Brandenburg U, Polzehl D, et al. Complement System in Healthy Term Newborns: Reference Values in Umbilical Cord Blood. Ped Develop Path 1998;1:131-5
Method(s):	1.	Single radial immunodiffusion (Binding Site, Birmingham, UK)
Comments:	1.	Studies were performed on cord blood obtained from 125 healthy term newborns. Results are 5-95th percentiles.

		Male and Female	
Test	**Age**	**n**	**mg/L**
1.	Term newborn cord blood	125	3.6 – 7.3
	>18y	31	2.7 – 5.4

COMPLEMENT FRACTION
Factor D

Specimen Type:	1	Plasma (EDTA or citrate)
Reference:	1.	Sonntag J, Brandenburg U, Polzehl D, et al. Complement System in Healthy Term Newborns: Reference Values in Umbilical Cord Blood. Ped Develop Path 1998;1:131-5
Method(s):	1.	Single radial immunodiffusion (Binding Site, Birmingham, UK)
Comments:	1.	Studies were performed on cord blood obtained from 125 healthy term newborns. Results are 5-95th percentiles.

COMPLEMENT FRACTION
Factor H

Test	Age	Male and Female	
		n	mg/L
1.	Term newborn cord blood	125	178 - 296
	>18y	31	146 - 553

Specimen Type:	1	Plasma (EDTA or citrate)
Reference:	1.	Sonntag J, Brandenburg U, Polzehl D, et al. Complement System in Healthy Term Newborns: Reference Values in Umbilical Cord Blood. Ped Develop Path 1998;1:131-5
Method(s):	1.	Single radial immunodiffusion (Binding Site, Birmingham, UK)
Comments:	1.	Studies were performed on cord blood obtained from 125 healthy term newborns. Results are 5-95th percentiles.

COMPLEMENT FRACTION
Factor I

| Test | Age | Male and Female | |
		n	mg/L
1.	Term newborn cord blood	125	15 - 32
	>18y	31	32 - 88

Specimen Type:	1	Plasma (EDTA or citrate)
Reference:	1.	Sonntag J, Brandenburg U, Polzehl D, et al. Complement System in Healthy Term Newborns: Reference Values in Umbilical Cord Blood. Ped Develop Path 1998;1:131-5
Method(s):	1.	Single radial immunodiffusion (Binding Site, Birmingham, UK)
Comments:	1.	Studies were performed on cord blood obtained from 125 healthy term newborns. Results are 5-95th percentiles.

COMPLEMENT FRACTION
Properdin

| Test | Age | Male and Female | |
		n	mg/L
1.	Term newborn cord blood	125	5.6 – 14.2
	>18y	31	24 - 50

Specimen Type:	1	Plasma (EDTA or citrate)
Reference:	1.	Sonntag J, Brandenburg U, Polzehl D, et al. Complement System in Healthy Term Newborns: Reference Values in Umbilical Cord Blood. Ped Develop Path 1998;1:131-5
Method(s):	1.	Single radial immunodiffusion (Binding Site, Birmingham, UK)
Comments:	1.	Studies were performed on cord blood obtained from 125 healthy term newborns. Results are 5-95th percentiles.

COPPER

Test	Age	n	Male µg/dL	Male µmol/L	n	Female µg/dL	Female µmol/L
1.	0 - 5d	27*	9 - 46	1.4 - 7.2	27*	9 - 46	1.4 - 7.2
	1 - 5y	77*	80 - 150	12.6 - 23.6	77*	80 - 150	12.6 - 23.6
	6 - 9y	44*	84 - 136	13.2 - 21.4	44*	84 - 136	13.2 - 21.4
	10 - 14y	36	80 - 121	12.6 - 19.0	23	82 - 120	12.9 - 18.9
	15 - 19y	55	64 - 171	10.1 - 18.4	31	72 - 160	11.3 - 25.2

Test	Age	n	Male and Female µg/dL	Male and Female µmol/L
2.	0 – <0.5y	13	38 – 104	5.9 – 16.3
	0.5 – <1.0y	18	24 – 152	3.8 – 23.8
	1.0 – <2.0y	15	76 – 193	11.9 – 30.3
	2.0 – <4.0y	23	87 – 187	13.7 – 29.3
	4.0 – <6.0y	19	56 – 191	8.8 – 30.0
	6.0 – <10.0y	25	117 – 181	18.4 – 28.4
	10.0 – <14.0y	21	87 – 182	13.7 – 28.5
	14.0 - <18.0y	17	75 – 187	11.7 – 29.3

Specimen Type:	1.	Serum
	2.	Serum/Plasma
Reference:	1.	Lockitch G, Halstead A, Wadsworth L, et al. Age and sex specific pediatric reference intervals for zinc, copper, selenium, iron, vitamins A and E and related proteins. Clin Chem 1988;34:1625-8.
	2.	Rükgauer M, Klein J, Kruse-Jarres J.D. Reference Values for the Trace Elements Copper, Manganese, Selenium, and Zinc in the Serum/Plasma of Children, Adolescents, and Adults. J. Trace Elements Med. Biol. 1997;11:92-8.
Method(s):	1.	Electrothermal Atomic absorption spectroscopy with deuterium background correction. Varian GTA-95 (Varian Canada, Inc., Mississauga, Canada).
	2.	Atomic Absorption Spectrophotometry with Zeeman background compensation Perkin Elmer ETAAS, Zeeman 3030, Uberlingen, Germany.
Comments:	1.	The study population was healthy children. Non-parametric methods were used to determine the 0.025 and 0.975 fractiles. *No significant differences were found for males and females. These ranges were therefore derived from combined data.
	2.	Study population was drawn from patients visiting the outpatient department or surgical or orthopedic ward for preoperative workup. Results are mean ± 2SDs. (2.5 – 97.5th percentiles)

CORTISOL

Test	Age	n	Male µg/L	nmol/L	n	Female µg/L	nmol/L
1.	5th day	*	6 - 198	17 - 546	*	6 - 198	17 - 546
	2 - 12mo	*	24 - 229	66 - 632	*	24 - 229	66 - 632
	2 - 13y	*	25 - 229	69 - 632	*	25 - 229	69 - 632
	14 - 15y	*	25 - 229	69 - 632	*	24 - 286	66 - 789
	16 - 18y	*	24 - 286	66 – 789	*	24 - 286	66 - 789
2.	5th day	*	6 - 156	16 – 431	*	6 – 156	16 – 431
	2 - 12mo	*	20 – 181	54 – 499	*	20 - 181	54 - 499
	2 - 13y	*	21 – 181	57 – 499	*	21 – 181	57 - 499
	14 – 15y	*	21 – 181	57 – 499	*	20 – 274	54 – 756
	16 – 18y	*	20 - 225	54 – 622	*	20 - 274	54 - 756

			Male and Female				
			5 – 11 am			5 – 11 pm	
		n	µg/L	nmol/L	n	µg/L	nmol/L
3.	0 - 24mo	33	10 – 340	28 – 938	25	10 – 300	28 – 828
	2 - <11y	31	10 – 330	28 – 911	23	10 – 240	28 – 662
	11 - 18y	31	10 - 280	28 – 773	19	10 - 220	28 - 607

Specimen Type:	1,2,3 Serum
Reference:	1. Jonetz-Mentzel L, Wiedemann G. Establishment of reference ranges for Cortisol in neonates, infants, children and adolescents. Eur J Clin Chem Biochem 1993;31:525-9.
	2. Murthy JN, Hicks JM, Soldin SJ. Evaluation of the Technicon Immuno I Random Access Immunoassay Analyzer and calculation of pediatric reference ranges for endocrine tests, T-uptake, and ferritin. Clin Biochem 1995;28:181-5
	3. Soldin SJ, Murthy JN, Agarwalla PK, et. al. Pediatric Reference Ranges for Creatine Kinase, CKMB, Troponin I, Iron and Cortisol. Clin Biochem 1999; 32:77-80.
Method(s):	1. TDx fluorescence polarization immunoassay. (Abbott Laboratories, Abbott Park, IL.)
	2. Bayer (Technicon) Immuno I analyzer with Bayer kits. (Bayer Corp., Tarrytown, NY.)
	3. Bayer Immuno I using Bayer Reagents. (Bayer Corp., Tarrytown, NY)
Comments:	1. 687 normal healthy neonates, infants, children and adolescents. Values are 2.5 to 97.5th percentiles. Results were rounded off to the nearest whole integer. *See reference for numbers.
	2. Results represent 2.5 - 97.5th percentiles. * n not given.
	3. Study used hospitalized patients and a computerized approach adapted from the Hoffman technic. Values are the 2.5-97.5th percentiles. Note that pm values are only moderately lower than am values.

C – REACTIVE PROTEIN (CRP)

Test	Age	n	Male and Female
			µg/L
1.	Cord serum	*	10 – 350
	Adult	*	68 – 8200
2.	Cord Serum	48	15 - 6000

Specimen Type:	1,2. Serum
Reference:	1. C. A. Burtis, C. R. Ashwood, Eds. Tietz Textbok of Clinical Chemistry. 2nd Edition. W.B. Saunders Co., 1994; 2184.
	2. Shine B, Gould J, Campbell C, et al. Serum C-reactive protein in normal and infected neonates. Clin Chim Acta 1985;148:97-103.
Method(s):	1. Nephelometric
Comments:	1. *Numbers not provided.
	2. 48 cord sera obtained from cord blood of normal neonates. Results are 5 – 95th percentiles. Values above 10,000 µg/L were found in neonates with infection.

CREATININE

Test	Age	n	mg/dL	µmol/L	Age	n	mg/dL	µmol/L
		Male			**Female**			
1.	0 - 1wk	*	0.6 - 1.1	53 - 97	0 - wk	*	0.6 - 1.1	53 - 97
	1wk - 1mo	*	0.3 - 0.7	27 - 62	1wk - 1mo	*	0.3 - 0.7	27 - 62
	1 - 6mo	*	0.2 - 0.4	18 - 35	1 - 6mo	*	0.2 - 0.4	18 - 35
	7 - 12mo	*	0.2 - 0.4	18 - 35	7m - 12mo	*	0.2 - 0.4	18 - 35
	1 - 18y	*	0.2 - 0.7	18 - 62	1 - 18y	*	0.2 - 0.7	18 - 62
2.	1 - 30d	42	0.5 - 1.2	44 - 106	1 - 30d	40	0.5 - 0.9	44 - 80
	31 - 365d	62	0.4 - 0.7	35 - 62	31 - 365d	59	0.4 - 0.6	35 - 53
	1 - 3y	103	0.4 - 0.7	35 - 62	1 - 3y	126	0.4 - 0.7	35 - 62
	4 - 6y	129	0.5 - 0.8	44 - 71	4 - 6y	116	0.5 - 0.8	44 - 71
	7 - 9y	121	0.6 - 0.9	53 - 80	7 - 9y	110	0.5 - 0.9	44 - 80
	10 - 12y	125	0.6 - 1.0	53 - 88	10 - 12y	117	0.6 - 1.0	53 - 88
	13 - 15y	135	0.6 - 1.2	53 - 106	13 - 15y	141	0.7 - 1.1	62 - 97
	16 - 18y	106	0.8 - 1.4	71 - 123	16 - 18y	114	0.8 - 1.2	71 - 106

Specimen Type: 1,2 Plasma

Reference:

1. Greeley C, Snell J, Colaco A, et al. Pediatric reference ranges for electrolytes and creatinine. Clin Chem 1993:39:1172. (Abstract)

2. Soldin SJ, Hicks JM, Bailey J, et al. Pediatric reference ranges for creatinine on the Hitachi 747 analyzer. Clin Chem 1997;43:S198. (Abstract)

Method(s):

1. Kodak Ektachem (Johnson & Johnson, Rochester, NY).

2. Jaffe method on Hitachi 747 Boehringer-Mannheim reagents. Boehringer-Mannheim Diagnostics, Indianapolis, IN.

Comments:

1. Study used hospitalized patients and a computerized approached to removing outliers.

   *N ≥ 100 in all of the above. Values are 2.5 - 97.5th percentiles.

2. Study used hospitalized patients and a computerized approach to removing outliers. Values reported are 2.5 - 97.5th percentiles.

CREATININE (URINE)

Age	n	Male and Female g/24h
3 - 8y	71	0.11 - 0.68
9 - 12y	45	0.17 - 1.41
13 - 17y	42	0.29 - 1.87
Adult	104	0.63 - 2.50

Specimen Type:	Urine
Reference:	Nichols Institute. Pediatric Endocrine Testing, 1993:35.
Method(s):	Kinetic, alkaline picrate.
Comments:	Results are 2.5 - 97.5th percentiles.

CREATINE KINASE

Test	Age	Male		Female	
		n	U/L	n	U/L
1.	0 – 90d	71	28 – 300	65	42 – 470
	3 – 12mo	129	24 - 170	90	26 - 240
	13 – 24mo	121	27 – 160	120	24 – 175
	2 - 10y	245	30 - 150	231	24 – 175
	11 – 14y	86	30 – 150	77	30 – 170
	15 - 18y	56	33 - 145	111	27 - 140
2.	1 - 30d	113	2 - 183	77	2 - 134
	31 – 182d	95	2 - 129	64	2 - 146
	183 – 365d	58	2 - 143	49	18 - 138
	1 - 3y	129	2 - 163	143	2 - 134
	4 - 6y	133	18 - 158	112	8 - 147
	7 - 9y	142	2 - 177	113	26 - 145
	10 - 12y	148	6 - 217	101	6 - 137
	13 - 15y	144	2 - 251	124	2 - 143
	16 - 18y	114	2 - 238	146	13 - 144

Specimen Type:	1,2	Plasma, Serum
Reference:	1.	Soldin SJ, Murthy JN, Agarwalla PK, et al. Pediatric Reference Ranges for Creatine Kinase, CKMB, Troponin I, Iron and Cortisol. Clin Biochem 1999;32:77-80.
	2.	Soldin SJ, Hicks JM, Bailey J, et al. Pediatric reference ranges for creatine kinase and insulin-like growth factor 1. Clin Chem 1997;43:S199. (Abstract)
Method(s):	1.	Ektachem 500 (Johnson & Johnson, Rochester NY). Creatine phosphate to creatine.
	2.	Hitachi 747 using Boehringer-Mannheim reagents. (Boehringer-Mannheim Diagnostics, Indianapolis, IN)
Comments:	1,2.	Study used hospitalized patients and a computerized adaptation of the Hoffmann technique. Values are 2.5 - 97.5th percentiles.

CREATINE KINASE ISOENZYMES
(CPK ISOENZYMES)

Test	Age	n	Male and Female	
			CKMB %	CKBB %
1.	Cord blood	*	0.3 - 3.1	0.3 - 10.5
	5 - 8h	*	1.7 - 7.9	3.6 - 13.4
	24 - 33h	*	1.8 - 5.0	2.3 - 8.6
	72 - 100h	*	1.4 - 5.4	5.1 - 13.3
	Adult	*	0 - 2.0	0

Test	Age	n	CKMB 97.5th percentile µg/L
2.	0 – 30d	76	4.5
	31 – 90d	45	4.8
	3 – 6mo	88	1.9
	7 – 12mo	47	1.7
	1 – 18y	97	1.7

Specimen Type:	1. Serum
	2. Serum/Plasma
Reference:	1. Behrman RE, Ed. Nelson textbook of pediatrics, 14th ed. Philadelphia, PA: WB Saunders Company, 1992:1807.
	2. Soldin SJ, Murthy JN, Agarwalla PK, et al. Pediatric Reference Ranges for Creatine Kinase, CKMB, Troponin I, Iron and Cortisol. Clin Biochem 1999;32:77-80.
Method(s):	1. Not provided.
	2. Bayer Immuno I with Bayer Reagents (Bayer Corp., Tarrytown, NY)
Comments:	1. *Numbers not given.
	2. Study used hospitalized patients and a computerized approach adapted from the Hoffmann technic. Values are the 97.5th percentiles.

DEHYDROEPIANDROSTERONE
(DHEA)

Test	Age	n	Male ng/dL	nmol/L	n	Female ng/dL	nmol/L
1.	6 - 9y	15	13 - 187	0.5 - 6.5	11	18 - 189	0.6 - 6.6
	10 - 11y	17	31 - 205	1.1 - 7.1	6	112 - 224	3.9 - 7.8
	12 - 14y	16	83 - 258	2.9 - 8.9	12	98 - 360	3.4 - 12.5
	Adults	*	180 - 1250	6.2 - 43.3	*	130 - 980	4.5 - 34.0
2.	0 – 1d	**	320 - 1100	11 - 39	**	460 - 1200	16 - 42
	1 - <7d	**	90 - 870	3 - 30	**	120 - 930	4 - 32
	7 - 28d	**	45 – 580	1.5 - 20	**	90 – 580	3 - 20
	1 – 12mo	**	9 – 290	0.3 – 10	**	17 – 170	0.6 - 6
	1 - <4y	**	12 – 90	0.4 - 3	**	20 - 45	0.7 – 1.6
	4 - 10y(P_1)	**	25 – 300	0.9 – 10	**	12 – 200	0.4 – 7.0
	P_2	**	50 – 580	1.8 – 20	**	60 – 1700	2 – 60
	P_3	**	130 – 640	4.5 – 22	**	125 – 1900	4.4 – 65
	P_4	**	190 – 730	6.5 – 25	**	170 – 1700	6 – 60
	P_5	**	230 – 730	8.0 – 25	**	220 – 810	7.5 – 28

Specimen Type:	1.	Serum
	2.	Plasma, Serum
Reference:	1.	Nichols Institute. Pediatric Endocrine Testing, 1993:13.
	2.	Soldin SJ, Rifai N, Hicks JM, Ed. *Biochemical Basis of Pediatric Disease* 3rd Edition. AACC Press, 1998; Chatper 9, 233.
Method(s):	1.	Extraction, Chromatography, Radioimmunoassay.
	2.	See reference
Comments:	1.	Results are 2.5 - 97.5th percentiles. *Numbers not provided.
	2.	**Numbers not provided. These reference ranges are for guidance only. P_1 – P_5 refer to pubertal stages.

DEHYDROEPIANDROSTERONE SULFATE
(DHEAS)

Test	Age	Male			Female		
		n	µg/dL	µmol/L	n	µg/dL	µmol/L
1.	0 - 1mo	56	9 - 316	0.2 - 8.6	41	15 - 261	0.4 - 7.1
	1 - 6mo	69	3 - 58	0.1 - 1.6	55	< 2 - 74	< 0.1 - 2.0
	7 - 12mo	40	< 2 - 26	< 0.1 - 0.7	28	< 2 - 26	< 0.1 - 0.7
	1 - 3y	114	< 2 - 15	< 0.1 - 0.4	121	< 2 - 22	< 0.1 - 0.6
	4 - 6y	95	< 2 - 27	< 0.1 - 0.7	86	< 2 - 34	< 0.1 - 0.9
	7 - 9y	103	< 2 - 60	< 0.1 - 1.6	83	< 2 - 74	< 0.1 - 2.0
	10 - 12y	95	5 - 137	0.1 - 3.7	55	3 - 111	0.1 - 3.0
	13 - 15y	86	3 - 188	0.1 - 5.1	78	4 - 171	0.1 - 4.6
	16 - 18y	62	26 - 189	0.7 - 5.1	69	10 - 237	0.3 - 6.4
2.	1 - 5mo	*	< 148	< 4	*	< 147	< 4
	6m - 7y	*	< 18	< 0.5	*	< 37	< 1.0
	8 - 9y	*	< 110	< 3	*	< 110	< 3
	10 - 12y	*	< 221	< 6	*	< 295	< 8
	13 - 19y	*	110 - 442	3 - 12	*	37 - 442	1 - 12

Specimen Type:	1.	Serum or Plasma
	2.	Serum
Reference:	1.	Soldin SJ, Godwin ID, Bailey J, et al. Pediatric reference ranges for DHEA sulfate. Clin Chem 1993;39:1171. (Abstract)
	2.	Babalola AA, Ellis G. Serum dehydroepiandrosterone sulfate in a normal pediatric population. Clin Biochem 1985;18:184-9.
Method(s):	1.	Diagnostic Product Corporation's Coat-a-Count DHEA-SO$_4$ procedure. (Diagnostic Products, Inc., Los Angeles CA.)
	2.	Used rabbit anti-DHA-3-hemisuccinyl-bovine-serum albumin antibody. (Radioimmunoassay, Inc., Toronto, Canada). Clin Biochem 1985;18:184-9.
Comments:	1.	Study used hospitalized patients and a computerized approach to removing outliers. Values are 2.5 - 97.5th percentiles.
	2.	Study used outpatients (131 boys and 143 girls) and provides the upper reference range.
		*See reference for appropriate numbers in each age interval.

DEOXYCORTICOSTERONE

Age	Male n	Male ng/dL	Female n	Female ng/dL
Prepubertal children	*	1 - 10	*	1 - 10
Adult	*	3.5 - 11.5		
Adult females				
follicular			*	1.5 - 8.5
luteal			*	3.5 - 13.0
Pregnancy				
1st trimester			*	5 - 25
2nd trimester			*	10 - 75
3rd trimester			*	30 - 110

Specimen Type:	Serum
Reference:	Nichols Institute. Pediatric Endocrine Testing, 1993:14
Method(s):	Extraction, Chromatography, Radioimmunoassay.
Comments:	Results are 2.5 - 97.5th percentiles.
	*Numbers not provided.

11-DEOXYCORTISOL
(COMPOUND S)

Age	n	Male and Female	
		µg/dL	nmol/L
6 - 9y	11	0.01 - 0.07	0.3 - 2.0
10 - 11y	17	0.01 - 0.09	0.3 - 2.6
12 - 14y	12	0.01 - 0.05	0.3 - 1.4
15 - 17y	10	0.02 - 0.05	0.6 - 1.4
Adult	*	≤ 0.12	≤ 3.5
Post metopirone reference range.	*	> 5.0	> 144

Specimen Type:	Serum
Reference:	Nichols Institute. Pediatric Endocrine Testing, 1993:14.
Method(s):	Extraction, Chromatography, Radioimmunoassay.
Comments:	Results are 2.5 - 97.5th percentiles.
	*Numbers not provided.

DOPAMINE (URINE)

Test	Age	n	Male and Female µg/g creatinine	Male and Female mmol/mol creatinine
1.	0 - 24mo	24	< 3,000	< 2.216
	2 - 4y	37	< 1,533	< 1.132
	5 - 9y	40	< 1,048	< 0.774
	10 - 19y	41	< 545	< 0.403
2.	< 1y	18	240 - 1,290	0.177 - 0.953
	1 - 4y	24	80 - 1,220	0.059 - 0.901
	4 - 10y	23	220 - 720	0.162 - 0.532
	10 - 18y	20	120 - 450	0.089 - 0.332

Specimen Type:	1,2	Urine
Reference:	1.	Soldin SJ, Lam G, Pollard A, et al. High performance liquid chromatographic analysis of urinary catecholamines employing amperometric detection: reference values and use in laboratory diagnosis of neural crest tumors. Clin Biochem 1980;13:285-91.
	2.	Rosano TG. Liquid chromatographic evaluation of age related changes in the urinary excretion of free catecholamines in pediatric patients. Clin Chem 1984;30:301-3.
Method(s):	1,2	HPLC with electrochemical detection.
Comments:	1.	Study involved healthy children. Results quoted are 95th percentile.
	2.	Urine was obtained from 85 pediatric patients (diagnosis of neoplasia excluded). Results are 0 - 100th percentiles.

EPINEPHRINE/ADRENALINE (PLASMA)

Test	Age	n	Male and Female	
			pg/mL	nmol/L
1.	2 - 10d	21	36 - 401	0.2 - 2.2
	10d - 3mo	10	55 - 201	0.3 - 1.1
	3 - 12mo	14	55 - 438	0.3 - 2.4
	12 - 24mo	13	36 - 639	0.2 - 3.5
	24 - 36mo	8	18 - 438	0.1 - 2.4
	36m - 15y	20	18 - 456	0.1 - 2.5
2.	30 min after birth	16	48 - 256	0.263 - 1.403
	2h after birth	16	92 - 140	0.504 - 0.767
	3h after birth	16	41 - 121	0.225 - 0.663
	12h after birth	16	8 - 12	0.044 - 0.066
	24h after birth	16	9 - 21	0.049 - 0.115
	48h after birth	16	18 - 34	0.099 - 0.186

Specimen Type:	1,2	Plasma
Reference:	1.	Candito M, Albertini M, Politano S, et al. Plasma catecholamine levels in children. J Chrom Biomed Appl 1993;617:304-7.
	2.	Eliot RJ, Lam R, Leake RD, et al. Plasma catecholamine concentrations in infants at birth and during the first 48 hours of life. J Pediatrics 1980;96:311-5.
Method(s):	1.	High performance liquid chromatography.
	2.	Radioenzymatic method.
Comments:	1.	Study population consisted of 86 healthy children (62 males, 24 females) aged 2 days to 15 years. Results are mean ± 2SD.
	2.	Study performed on 16 term vaginally delivered infants. Results are mean ± 2SD.

EPINEPHRINE/ADRENALINE (URINE)

Test	Age	Male and Female		
		n	μg/g creatinine	mmol/mol creatinine
1.	0 - 24mo	24	< 75	< 0.046
	2 - 4y	37	< 57	< 0.035
	5 - 9y	40	< 35	< 0.022
	10 - 19y	41	< 34	< 0.021
2.	0 - 12mo	18	0 - 375	0 - 0.232
	1 - 4y	24	0 - 82	0 - 0.051
	4 - 10y	22	5 - 93	0.003 - 0.057
	10 - 18y	20	3 - 58	0.001 - 0.027

Specimen Type:	1,2 Urine
Reference:	1. Soldin SJ, Lam G, Pollard A, et al. High performance liquid chromatographic analysis of urinary catecholamines employing amperometric detection: Reference values and use in laboratory diagnosis of neural crest tumors. Clin Biochem 1980;13:285-91.
	2. Rosano TG. Liquid chromatographic evaluation of age related changes in the urinary excretion of free catecholamines in pediatric patients. Clin Chem 1984;30:301-3.
Method(s):	1,2 HPLC with electrochemical detection.
Comments:	1. Study involved healthy children. Results quoted are 95th percentile.
	2. Urine was obtained from 85 pediatric patients. (Patients with a discharge diagnosis of neoplasia, endocrinopathy, or muscular dystrophy were not included in the study.) Results are 0 - 100th percentiles.

ERYTHROPOIETIN

Age	Male		Female	
	n	mIU/mL	n	mIU/mL
1 - 3y	122	1.7 - 17.9	97	2.1 - 15.9
4 - 6y	89	3.5 - 21.9	76	2.9 - 8.5
7 - 9y	79	1.0 - 13.5	80	2.1 - 8.2
10 - 12y	98	1.0 - 14.0	90	1.1 - 9.1
13 - 15y	100	2.2 - 14.4	148	3.8 - 20.5
16 - 18y	66	1.5 - 15.2	77	2.0 - 14.2

Specimen Type:	Plasma
Reference:	Krafte-Jacobs B, Williams J, Soldin SJ. Plasma erythropoietin reference ranges in children. J Pediatrics 1995;126:601-3.
Method(s):	ELISA (Quantikine™ IVD™, Human EPO Immunoassay [R and D Systems, Minneapolis, MN.])
Comments:	Study used hospitalized patients and a computerized approach to removing outliers. Values are 2.5 - 97.5th percentiles.

ESTRADIOL

Test	Age	Male			Female		
		n	pg/mL	pmol/L	n	pg/mL	pmol/L
1.	0 - 30d	38	8.0 – 53.0	29 - 194	22	12.0 – 66.0	44 – 241.6
	31 - 182d	51	1.0 – 12.0	3.7 - 44	31	1.0 – 11.0	3.7 – 40.3
	6mo – 3y	116	0.3 – 6.1	1.1 – 22.3	100	0.4 – 7.9	1.5 – 28.9
	4 - 6y	43	0.9 – 5.5	3.3 – 20.1	27	1.8 – 8.3	6.6 – 30.4
	7 - 9y	40	0.3 – 9.6	1.1 – 35.1	18	1.3 – 7.4	4.8 – 27.1
	10 - 12y	43	0.4 – 10.0	1.5 – 36.6	27	0.3 –20.6	1.1 – 75.4
	13 - 15y	33	0.5 – 9.6	1.8 – 35.1	39	0.3 – 33.2	1.1 – 121.5
	16 - 18y	14	3.6 – 20.4	13.2 – 74.7	24	4.4 – 49.2	16.1 – 180.1
2.	1 - 6y	**	< 15	< 55	**	< 15	< 55
	7 - 10y	**	< 15	< 55	**	< 70	< 257
	11 - 12y	**	< 40	< 147	**	10 - 300	37 - 1100
	13 - 15y	**	< 45	< 165	**	10 - 300	37 - 1100
	16 - 17y	**	10 - 50	37 – 184	**	10 - 300	37 - 1100

Specimen Type:	1. Serum/Plasma 2. Plasma
Reference:	1. Soldin SJ, Hicks JM, Bailey J, et al. Pediatric Reference Ranges for Estradiol and C1 Esterase Inhibitor. Clin Chem 1998; 44:A17. (Abstract) 2. Adaptation of method of Abraham GE, Odell WD, Swerdloff RS, et al. Simultaneous radioimmunoassay of plasma FSH, LH, progester-one, 17-hydroxy-progesterone and estradiol-17 beta during the menstrual cycle. J Clin Endocrinol Metab 1972;34:312-8. Meites S, Ed. Pediatric clinical chemistry, 3rd ed. Washington, DC: AACC Press, 1989:122-3.
Method(s):	1. Immunoassay. ACS 180 using Chiron reagents (Chiron Diagnostics Corp. East Walpole, MA) 2. Extraction followed by RIA.
Comments:	1. The study used serum/plasma from hospitalized patients and employed Chauvenet's criteria for removing outliers and a computerized approach adapted from the Hoffmann technic to obtain the 2.5 – 97.5[th] percentiles. 2. **See pp. 122-3 of *Pediatric Clinical Chemistry* for numbers.

FERRITIN

Test	Age	Male			Female		
		n	ng/mL	µg/L	n	ng/mL	µg/L
1.	1 - 5y*	44	6 - 24	6 - 24	44	6 - 24	6 - 24
	6 - 9y*	50	10 - 55	10 - 55	50	10 - 55	10 - 55
	10 - 14y	31	23 - 70	23 - 70	40	6 - 40	6 - 40
	14 - 19y	65	23 - 70	23 - 70	110	6 - 40	6 - 40
2.	1 - 30d	83	6 - 400	6 - 400	66	6 - 515	6 - 515
	1 - 6mo	70	6 - 410	6 - 410	50	6 - 340	6 - 340
	7 - 12mo	51	6 - 80	6 - 80	51	6 - 45	6 - 45
	1 - 5y	82	6 - 60	6 - 60	90	6 - 60	6 - 60
	6 - 19y	77	6 - 320	6 - 320	121	6 - 70	6 - 70
3.	1 - 30d	83	36 - 381	36 - 381	66	36 - 483	36 - 483
	1 - 6mo	70	36 - 391	36 - 391	50	36 - 329	36 - 329
	7 - 12mo	51	36 - 100	36 - 100	51	36 - 70	36 - 70
	1 - 5y	82	36 - 84	36 - 84	90	36 - 84	36 - 84
	6 - 19y	77	36 - 311	36 - 311	121	36 - 92	36 - 92

Specimen Type:	1,2,3 Plasma, Serum
Reference:	1. Lockitch G, Halstead A, Wadsworth L, et al. Age and sex specific pediatric reference intervals for zinc, copper, selenium, iron, vitamins A and E and related proteins. Clin Chem 1988;34:1625-8.
	2. Soldin SJ, Morales A, Albalos F, et al. Pediatric reference ranges on the Abbott IMx for FSH, LH, prolactin, TSH, T4, T3, free T4, Free T3, T-uptake, and ferritin. Clin Biochem 1995;28:603-6.
	3. Murthy JN, Hicks JM, Soldin SJ. Evaluation of the Technicon Immuno I Random Access Immunoassay Analyzer and calculation of pediatric reference ranges for endocrine tests, T-uptake, and ferritin. Clin Biochem 1995;28:181-5.
Method(s):	1. Ferritin was measured by immunoassay and using ferrizyme reagent (Abbott Laboratories, Abbott Park, IL).
	2. IMx analyzer (Abbott Laboratories, Abbott Park, IL).
	3. Bayer Immuno I with Bayer reagents (Bayer Corp., Tarrytown NY).
Comments:	1. The study population was healthy children. Non-parametric methods were used to determine the 0.025 and 0.975 fractiles.
	*No significant differences were found for males and females. These ranges were therefore derived from combined data.
	2, 3 Study used hospitalized patients and a computerized approach adapted from the Hoffmann technique. Values are 2.5 - 97.5th percentiles.
	Note: Ferritin levels of < 6 µg/L are strongly suggestive of iron deficiency.

FOLIC ACID

Test	Age	Male n	Male nmol/L	Female n	Female nmol/L
1.	0 - 1y	111	16.3 - 50.8	73	14.3 - 51.5
	2 - 3y	105	5.7 - 34.0	135	3.9 - 35.6
	4 - 6y	154	1.1 - 29.4	104	6.1 - 31.9
	7 - 9y	103	5.2 - 27.0	102	5.4 - 30.4
	10 - 12y	105	3.4 - 24.5	90	2.3 - 23.1
	13 - 18y	127	2.7 - 19.9	159	2.7 - 16.3
2.	Newborn[a]	*	16 - 72	*	16 - 72
	After newborn period	*	4 - 20	*	4 - 20
	Adult[a,b,c]	*	10 - 63	*	10 - 63

Specimen Type:	1. Plasma 2. Serum
Reference:	1. Hicks JM, Cook J, Godwin ID, et al. Vitamin B_{12} and folate: pediatric reference ranges. Arch Pathol Lab Med, 1993;117:704-6. 2. a. Behrman RE, Vaughan VC, Eds. Nelson textbook of pediatrics. Philadelphia, PA: WB Saunders Company 1983:1827-60. b. Nathan DG, Oski FA. Hematology of infancy and childhood, 4th ed. Appendix IX. Philadelphia, PA: WB Saunders Company, 1993. c. Hall CA, Bardwell SA, Allen ES, et al. Variation in plasma folate levels among groups of healthy persons. Am J Clin Nutr 1975;28:854-7.
Method(s):	1. Radioimmunoassay Quantaphase (BioRad, Hercules, CA). 2. See references.
Comments:	1. Study used hospitalized patients and a computerized approach adapted from the Hoffmann technique to obtain the 2.5 - 97.5th percentiles. 2. *See references for particulars of assays used and numbers studied.

FOLLICLE STIMULATING HORMONE
(FSH)

Test	Age	Male		Female	
		n	U/L	n	U/L
1.	< 2y	110	0.2 - 1.8	33	0.2 - 6.6
	2 - 5y	124	0.2 - 1.4	96	0.2 - 3.8
	6 - 10y	99	0.2 - 1.3	155	0.2 - 2.7
	11 - 20y	100	0.2 - 8.0	247	0.2 - 8.0
2.	< 2y	110	0.4 - 2.1	33	0.4 - 7.1
	2 - 5 y	124	0.4 - 1.7	94	0.4 - 4.2
	6 - 10y	99	0.4 - 1.6	136	0.4 - 3.0
	11 - 20y	100	0.4 - 8.7	263	0.4 - 8.6

Specimen Type:	1,2	Plasma or serum.
Reference:	1.	Soldin SJ, Morales A, Albalos F, et al. Pediatric reference ranges on the Abbott IMx for FSH, LH, prolactin, TSH, T_4, T_3, free T_4, free T_3, T-uptake, IgE and ferritin. Clin Biochem 1995;28:603-6.
	2.	Murthy JN, Hicks JM, Soldin SJ. Evaluation of the Technicon Immuno I Random Access Immunoassay Analyzer and calculation of pediatric reference ranges for endocrine tests, T-uptake, and ferritin. Clin Biochem 1995;28:181-5.
Method(s):	1.	IMx (Abbott Laboratories, Abbott Park, IL).
	2.	Technicon Immuno I with Bayer reagents (Bayer Corp., Tarrytown, NY).
Comments:	1,2	Study used hospitalized patients and a computerized approach to removing outliers. Values are 2.5 - 97.5th percentiles.

FREE FATTY ACIDS

Age	n	Male and Female
		mmol/L
1 - 12mo	12	0.5 - 1.6
1 - 7mo	27	0.6 - 1.5
7 - 15y	9	0.2 - 1.1

Specimen Type:	Plasma
Reference:	Bonnefont JP, Specola NB, Vassault A, et al. The fasting test in pediatrics: application to the diagnosis of pathological hypo- and hyperketotic states. Eur J Pediatr 1990;150:80-5.
Method(s):	Standard enzymatic procedure. See reference.
Comments:	Results are 10 - 90th percentiles.

FRUCTOSAMINE

Test	Age	Male and Female	
		n	mmol/L
1.	0 – 3y	33	1.56 - 2.27
	3 – 6y	49	1.73 - 2.34
	6 – 9y	35	1.82 - 2.56
	9 – 12y	24	2.04 - 2.50
	12 – 15y	29	2.02 - 2.63
2.	Normal	203	0.174 - 0.286
	Controlled Diabetics	80	0.210 - 0.421
	Uncontrolled Diabetics	123	0.268 - 0.870

Specimen Type:	1,2	Serum
Reference:	1.	De Schepper J, Derde MP, Goubert P, et al. Reference values for fructosamine concentrations in children's sera: influence of protein concentration, age and sex. Clin Chem 1988;34:2444-7.
	2.	RoTAG™ Fructosamine (Glycated Protein) Assay from package insert Roche diagnostics kit.
Method(s):	1.	Roche diagnostics kit on Cobas-Bio (Roche Diagnostic Systems, Inc., Branchburg, NJ).
	2.	Roche diagnostics kit (Roche Diagnostic Systems, Inc., Branchburg, NJ).
Comments:	1.	Results are 2.5 - 97.5th percentiles.
	2.	Results using the new Roche kit using polylysine differ by a factor of approximately 10 from the old kit using DMF equivalents. Ages not provided in study.

GAMMA-GLUTAMYLTRANSFERASE
(GGT)

Test	Age	Male n	Male U/L	Female n	Female U/L
1.	1 - 182d	109	12 – 122	67	15 – 132
	183 - 365d	36	1 – 39	36	1 – 39
	1 - 12y	488	3 – 22	391	4 – 22
	13 - 18y	170	2 – 42	208	4 – 24
2.**	1 - 7d	137	25 – 148	102	19 – 131
	8 - 30d	186	23 – 153	129	17 – 124
	1 - 3mo	172	17 – 130	189	17 – 124
	4 - 6mo	241	8 – 83	191	15 – 109
	7 - 12mo	199	10 – 35	190	10 – 54
3.**	1 - 3y	50*	5 – 16	50*	5 – 16
	4 - 6y	40*	8 – 18	40*	8 – 18
	7 - 9y	80*	11 – 21	80*	11 – 21
	10 - 11y	27	14 – 25	34	14 – 23
	12 - 13y	31	14 – 37	49	12 – 21
	14 - 15y	26	10 – 28	52	12 – 22
	16 - 19y	40	9 – 29	61	9 – 23

Specimen Type:
1, 2 Serum or Plasma
3. Plasma

Reference:

1. Soldin SJ, Hicks JM, Bailey J, et al. Pediatric reference ranges for gamma-glutamyltransferase. Clin Chem 1997;43:S198. (Abstract)

2. Soldin SJ, Savwoir TV, Guo Y. Pediatric reference ranges for gamma-glutamyltransferase and urea nitrogen during the first year of life on the Vitros 500 analyzer. Clin Chem 1997;43:S199. (Abstract)

3. Lockitch G, Halstead AC, Albersheim S, et al. Age and sex specific pediatric reference intervals for biochemistry analytes as measured with the Ektachem 700 analyzer. Clin Chem 1988;34:1622-5.

Method(s):

1. Substrate used is L-α-glutamyl-3-carboxy-4-nitroanilide and rate of production of 5-amino-2-nitrobenzoate is measured on the Hitachi 747. Boehringer-Mannheim Reagents (Boehringer-Mannheim Diagnostics, Indianapolis, IN).

2, 3 Ektachem 500 (2) and 700 (3) (Johnson & Johnson, Rochester, NY). α-glutamyl-p-nitroanilide used as substrate.

Comments:

1, 2 Study used hospitalized patients and a computerized approach adapted from the Hoffmann technique. Values are 2.5 - 97.5th percentiles.

3. The study population was healthy children. Non-parametric methods were used to determine the 0.025 and 0.975 fractiles.

*Males and females were not studied separately.

** The values originally published were multiplied by 0.8383 to accommodate changes made by the manufacturer which decreased values by approx. 16%.

GASTRIN		
		Male and Female
Age	**n**	**ng/L** **pg/mL**
Newborns (1 - 12d)	*	69 - 190
Infants (1.5 - 22mo)	*	55 - 186
Prepubertal and pubertal children fasting 3 - 4h	*	2 - 168
5 - 6h	*	3 - 117
≥ 8h	*	1 - 125

Specimen Type:	Serum
Reference:	Nichols Institute. Pediatric Endocrine Testing, 1993:20.
Method(s):	Radioimmunoassay
Comments:	Results are 2.5 - 97.5th percentiles. *See reference for numbers.

GLOBULINS
TOTAL, CALCULATED

Test	Age	Male			Female		
		n	g/dL	g/L	n	g/dL	g/L
1.	1 - 182d	58	1.3 - 2.4	13 - 24	51	1.3 - 2.1	13 - 24
	183 - 365d	29	1.7 - 3.0	17 - 30	42	1.2 - 2.4	12 - 24
	1 - 3y	134	2.1 - 3.4	21 - 34	186	1.8 - 3.3	18 - 33
	4 - 6y	139	2.2 - 3.4	22 - 34	114	2.0 - 3.6	20 - 36
	7 - 9y	118	2.2 - 3.6	22 - 36	107	2.2 - 3.4	22 - 34
	10 - 12y	89	2.4 - 3.4	24 - 34	82	2.3 - 3.3	23 - 33
	13 - 15y	97	2.1 - 3.7	21 - 37	83	2.4 - 3.8	24 - 38
	16 - 18y	75	2.0 - 3.9	20 - 39	54	2.6 - 3.6	26 - 36
2.	< 1y	104*	0.4 - 3.7	4 - 37	104*	0.4 - 3.7	4 - 37
	1 - 3y	247*	1.6 - 3.5	16 - 35	247*	1.6 - 3.5	16 - 35
	4 - 9y	694*	1.9 - 3.4	19 - 34	694*	1.9 - 3.4	19 - 34
	10 - 49y	17,905*	1.9 - 3.5	19 - 35	17,905*	1.8 - 3.5	18 - 35

Specimen Type:	1.	Plasma
	2.	Serum
Reference:	1.	Hicks JM, Bjorn S, Beatey J, et al. Pediatric reference ranges for albumin, globulin and total protein on the Hitachi 747. Clin Chem 1995;41:S93 (Abstract).
	2.	Appleton C. Queensland Medical Laboratory, Brisbane, Australia. Meites, S, Ed. Pediatric clinical chemistry, 3rd ed. Washington, DC: AACC Press, 1989:132.
Method(s):	1.	Calculated (Total Protein - Albumin).
	2.	Calculated. Obtained by subtracting albumin values from total protein values obtained on the Technicon SMAC II Analyzer (Technicon Instruments Corp., Tarrytown, NY).
Comments:	1.	Study used hospitalized patients and a computerized approach adapted from the Hoffmann technique. Values are 2.5 - 97.5th percentiles.
	2.	Values are 2.5 - 97.5th percentiles.
		*Numbers listed include males and females.

GLUCAGON

Age	n	Male and Female ng/L pg/mL
Cord blood	6	0 - 215
3d	12	0 - 1750
4 - 14y	9	0 - 148

Specimen Type:	Plasma
Reference:	Nichols Institute. Pediatric Endocrine Testing, 1993:20.
Method(s):	Extraction, Radioimmunoassay.
Comments:	Results are 2.5 - 97.5th percentiles.

GLUCOSE

Test	Age	Male and Female		
		n	mg/dL	mmol/L
1.	0 – 1mo	207	55 - 115	3.1 - 6.4
	1 – 6mo	96	57 - 117	3.2 - 6.5
2.	Outside the neonatal period	482*	70 - 126	3.9 - 7.0

Specimen Type:	1. Whole blood. 2. Serum
Reference:	1. Snell J, Greeley C, Colaco A, et al. Pediatric reference ranges for arterial pH whole blood electrolytes and glucose. Clin Chem 1993;39:1173. (Abstract) 2. Lockitch G, Halstead AC, Albersheim S, et al. Age and sex specific pediatric reference intervals for biochemistry analyses as measured with the Ektachem 700 analyzer. Clin Chem 1988;34:1622-5.
Method(s):	1. Glucose oxidase YSI 2300 (Yellow Springs Instruments, Yellow Springs, OH). 2. Glucose oxidase, Kodak Ektachem 700 (Johnson & Johnson, Rochester, NY).
Comments:	1. Results are 2.5 - 97.5th percentiles. The 0 - 1mo group includes an appreciable number of premature infants. 2. Results are 2.5 - 97.5th percentiles. *No significant differences were found for males and females. These ranges were therefore derived from combined data.

GLUCOSE CEREBROSPINAL FLUID
(CSF GLUCOSE)

Age	n	Male and Female
All ages	*	60 - 80% of blood glucose

Specimen Type:	Cerebrospinal fluid
Reference:	Meites S, Ed. Pediatric clinical chemistry, 2nd ed. Washington, DC: AACC Press, 1981:216-8.
Comments:	Glucose is measured in CSF primarily in the diagnosis of bacterial meningitis. CSF glucose should be compared to blood glucose for interpretation. *Number not provided.

GLUTATHIONE PEROXIDASE ACTIVITY

Age	n	Male and Female
		U/L
Newborn (term)	*	180 - 890
1 - 5y	*	554 - 985
6 - 15y	*	567 - 1153
16 y - adult	*	780 - 1269

Specimen Type:	Serum
Reference:	Lockitch G. Trace elements in pediatrics. JIFCC 1996:9; 46-51.
Method(s):	Enzymatic
Comments:	*Numbers of individuals included in each age range not provided. In selenium deficiency activity of glutathione peroxidase in plasma/serum reflects selenium status.

GROWTH HORMONE

Test	Age	n	Male and Female μg/L
1.	5 - 10y	24	> 3*
	11.7 - 15.5y	14	> 3.9*
	5 - 10y	24	5.7 ± 0.6**
	11.7 - 15.5y	14	6.2 ± 0.7**
	5 - 10y	24	≥ 20***
	11.7 - 15.5y	14	≥ 20***
2.	After stimulation by exercise, arginine or insulin		> 5

Specimen Type:	1. Plasma 2. Serum
Reference:	1. Dammacco F, Boghen MF, Camanni F, et al. Somatotropic function in short stature: evaluation by integrated auxological and hormonal indices in 214 children. J Clin Endocrinol Metab, 1993:77;68-72. 2. Reference values and SI unit information. The Hospital for Sick Children, Toronto, Canada, 1993:369.
Method(s):	1. Immunoradiometric assay (Sorin, Saluggia, Italy). 2. RIA.
Comments:	1. *overnight minimal GH concentration. **overnight mean GH concentration ± SEM. ***Responsiveness to stimulation with GH releasing hormone and pyridostigmine. 2. Differential diagnosis of short stature, slow growth or evaluation of pituitary function. Random samples have little diagnostic value.

GROWTH HORMONE (URINE)

Test	Age	Male			Female		
		n	ng/24h	ng/g creatinine	n	ng/24h	ng/g creatinine
1.	2.2-13.3y Tanner 1	*	0.4 - 6.3	0.9 - 12.3	*	0.4 - 6.3	0.9 - 12.3
	10.3-14.6y Tanner 2	*	0.8 - 12.0	1.0 - 14.1	*	0.8 - 12.0	1.0 - 14.1
	11.5-15.3y Tanner 3	*	1.7 - 20.4	1.9 - 17.0	*	1.7 - 20.4	1.9 - 17.0
	12.7-17.1y Tanner 4	*	1.5 - 18.2	1.3 - 14.4	*	1.5 - 18.2	1.3 - 14.4
	13.5-19.9y Tanner 5	*	1.2 - 14.5	0.8 - 11.0	*	1.2 - 14.5	0.8 - 11.0
	Adults	*	0.6 - 20.9	0.4 - 15.9	*	0.6 - 20.9	0.4 - 15.9
2.	3 - 4y	**		> 6.5	**		> 9.1
	5 - 6y	**		> 8.7	**		> 8.9
	7 - 8y	**		> 6.8	**		> 5.9
	9 - 10y	**		> 5.6	**		> 8.9
	11 - 12y	**		> 6.2	**		> 9.3
	13 - 14y	**		> 10.5	**		> 6.3
	15 - 16y	**		> 3.8	**		> 5.1
	17 - 18y	**		> 3.1	**		> 3.1
	19 - 20y	**		> 1.9	**		> 1.9

Specimen Type:	1, 2 Urine
Reference:	1. Main K, Philips M, Jergensen M, et al. Urinary growth hormone excretion in 657 healthy children and adults. Normal values, inter- and intraindividual variations. Horm Res 1991;36:174-82 2. Nukada O, Moriwake T, Kanzaki S, et al. Age-related changes in urinary growth hormone level and its clinical application. Acta Paediatr Jpn 1990;32:32-8.
Method(s):	1. Elisa, antipituitary hGH (Nanormon® and recombinant hGH (Norditropin®). (Novo Nordisk A/S, Gentofte, Denmark). 2. EIA (Sumitomo Chemical Co., Ltd., Takarazuka, Japan).
Comments:	1. 547 healthy children and 110 *See reference for numbers healthy adults. Results are 2.5 - 97.5th percentiles.. 2. Study evaluated urinary GH secretion in 270 normal subjects aged 3 - 20 years. Results provided are the *lower* limit of normal (Mean - 2SD). **See reference for numbers.

HEMOGLOBIN A₁c

Test	Age	n	%
		Male and Female	
1.	Normal individuals	*	4 - 7
	Pregnant women	*	5 - 8
	Old age	*	6 - 9
	Stable diabetics	*	8 - 10
	Young or unstable diabetics	*	8 - 18
2.	Normal individuals	**	3.4 - 6.1
3.	Healthy non-diabetics	***	4 - 6
	Diabetics with average control	***	9 - 10

Specimen Type:	1,2,3 Whole blood.
Reference:	1. Kellen JA. Disorders of carbohydrate metabolism. In: AG Gornall, Ed. Applied biochemistry of clinical disorders, 2nd ed. Philadelphia, PA: J.B. Lippincott Company, 1986:379-402.
	2. Children's National Medical Center, Washington, DC. Unpublished data.
	3. Reference values and SI unit information. The Hospital for Sick Children, Toronto, Canada, 1993.
Method(s):	1. Not provided.
	2. Immunochemical technique DCA 2000 Hemoglobin A₁C System. (Miles Diagnostics Division, Elkhart, IN.)
	3. High-performance liquid chromatography.
Comments:	1. *Numbers are not provided.
	2. **Numbers are not provided. Hemoglobin is glycated in proportion to the average blood glucose concentration over the life span of the red cell (90 - 120d). Hemoglobin A₁c allows tracking of metabolic control in individual patients over time.
	3. ***Numbers not provided.

101

HIGH-DENSITY LIPOPROTEIN CHOLESTEROL
(HDL CHOLESTEROL)

Test	Age	n	mg/dL	mmol/L	n	mg/dL	mmol/L
			Male			**Female**	
1.	1 - 9y	50*	35 - 82	0.91 - 2.12	50*	35 - 82	0.91 - 2.12
	10 - 13y	56*	36 - 84	0.93 - 2.17	56*	36 - 84	0.93 - 2.17
	14 - 19y	60*	35 - 65	0.91 - 1.68	60*	35 - 65	0.91 - 1.68
2.	5y	**	37 - 72	0.96 - 1.86	**	34 - 69	0.88 - 1.78
	10y	**	31 - 70	0.80 - 1.81	**	34 - 69	0.88 - 1.78
	15y	**	29 - 61	0.75 - 1.58	**	34 - 69	0.88 - 1.78
	20y	**	29 - 58	0.75 - 1.50	**	36 - 70	0.93 - 1.81
3.	0 – 24mo	43 *	8 - 61	0.21 – 1.58	43*	8 - 61	0.21 – 1.58
	2 - <7y	95	23 – 70	0.60 - 1.81	71	12 – 64	0.31 - 1.66
	7 - <12y	99	25 - 79	0.65 – 2.05	133	23 - 80	0.60 – 2.07
	12 - <16y	199	19 – 76	0.49 – 1.97	181	25 – 83	0.65 – 2.15
	16 - <19y	91	26 - 75	0.67 – 1.94	157	21 - 77	0.54 – 1.99

102

Specimen Type:	1.	Serum
	2.	Plasma
	3.	Serum/Plasma
Reference:	1.	Lockitch G, Halstead AC, Albersheim S, et al. Age and sex specific pediatric reference intervals for biochemistry analytes as measured with the Ektachem 700 analyzer. Clin Chem 1988;34:1622-5.
	2.	Kottke BA, Moll PP, Michels VV, et al. Levels of lipids, lipoproteins and apolipoproteins in a defined population. Mayo Clin Proc 1991;66:1198-1208.
	3.	Murthy JN, Soldin SJ. Pediatric Reference Ranges for HDL-Cholesterol on the Vitros 500 Anlayzer. Clin Chem 1999; 45; A23. (Abstract)
Method(s):	1, 3.	Dextran sulfate precipitation/cholesterol oxidase. Kodak Ektachem 700 (1) and 500 (3) (Johnson & Johnson, Rochester, NY).
	2.	LDL and VLDL precipitated using polyethylene glycol 6000. Supernatant used to determine HDL-cholesterol by an enzymatic method. See reference.
Comments:	1.	Healthy children. Results are 2.5 - 97.5th percentiles.
		*No significant differences were found for males and females. These ranges were therefore derived from combined data.
	2.	Results are 5 - 95th percentiles read off graphs in reference.
		**See reference for numbers.
	3.	* Male and Female combined. The study used hospitalized patients and employed Chauvenet's criteria for removing outliers and a computerized approach adapted from the Hoffmann technic to obtain the 2.5 – 97.5th percentiles. The 2.5th and 97.5th percentiles are lower during the first 2y of life. For children >2y, the 2.5th percentiles are lower than those previously described by Lockitch et al Clin Chem 1988; 34:1622-5

HOMOCYSTEINE (TOTAL)

Age	n	Male and Female
		µmol/L
2mo - 10y	105	3.3 - 8.3
11 - 15y	59	4.7 - 10.3
16 - 18y	31	4.7 - 11.3

Specimen Type:	Plasma
Reference:	Vilaseca MA, Moyano D, Ferrer I, et al. Total homocysteine in pediatric patients. Clin Chem 1997;43:690-2.
Method(s):	HPLC
Comments:	This study was performed on plasma obtained from healthy children. Results are the 2.5th and 97.5th percentiles.

HOMOVANILLIC ACID (HVA)
4-HYDROXY-3-METHOXYPHENYLACETIC ACID (URINE)

Test	Age	n	mg/g creatinine	mmol/mol creatinine	n	mg/24h	μmol/24h
			Male and Female				
1.	0 - 1y	37	< 32.6	< 20.2	48	< 2.8	< 15.4
	2 - 4y	49	< 22.0	< 13.6	34	< 4.7	< 25.8
	5 - 9y	79	< 15.1	< 9.4	20	< 5.4	< 29.6
	10 - 19y	55	< 12.8	< 7.9	40	< 7.2	< 39.5
	> 19y	56	< 7.6	< 4.7	56	< 8.3	< 45.6
2.	0 - 3mo	12	11.3 - 35.0	7.0 - 21.7			
	3 - 12mo	30	8.4 - 44.9	5.2 - 27.8			
	1 - 2y	16	12.2 - 31.8	7.6 - 19.7			
	2 - 5y	21	3.4 - 32.0	2.1 - 19.8			
	5 - 10y	25	6.8 - 23.7	4.2 - 14.7			
	10 - 15y	13	3.2 - 13.6	2.0 - 8.4			
	> 15y	9	3.2 - 9.6	2.0 - 6.0			

Specimen Type: 1,2 Urine

Reference:

1. Soldin SJ, Hill JG. Liquid chromatographic analysis for urinary 4-hydroxy-3-methoxy-mandelic acid and 4-hydroxy-3-methoxy-phenylacetic acid and its use in investigation of neural crest tumors. Clin Chem 1981;27:502-3.

2. Tuchman M, Morris CL, Ramnaraine ML, et al. Value of random urinary homovanillic acid and vanillyl mandelic acid levels in the diagnosis and management of patients with neuroblastoma: comparison with 24-hour urine collections. Pediatrics 1985;75: 324-8.

Method(s):

1. HPLC with electrochemical detection.
2. Capillary gas chromatography.

Comments:

1. Analysis performed on patients under investigation of hypertension or not suspected of having a neural crest tumor. All patients studied free of neoplasia. Results are 95th percentile.

2. Values are 0 - 100th percentiles. Normal values were obtained from 93 pediatric patients in whom the diagnosis of neural crest tumors had been excluded.

HYALURONIC ACID

Age	n	Male and Female
		µg/L
1 - 3mo	*	49 - 153
2 - 3y	*	9 - 40
4 - 18y	*	6 - 32

Specimen Type:	Serum
Reference:	Trivedi P, Cheeseman P, Mowat AP. Serum hyaluronic acid in healthy infants and children and its value as a marker of progressive hepatobiliary disease starting in infancy. Clin Chim Acta 1993;215:29-39.
Method(s):	Affinity-binding radiometric assay (Pharmacia Diagnostics AB, Uppsala, Sweden).
Comments:	397 healthy infants. *See reference for details.

β-HYDROXYBUTYRATE
3-HYDROXYBUTYRATE

Age	n	Male and Female	
		mg/dL	mmol/L
1 - 12mo	12	1.0 - 10.0	0.1 - 1.0
1 - 7y	27	< 1.0 - 9.4	< 0.1 - 0.9
7 - 15y	9	< 1.0 - 3.1	< 0.1 - 0.3

Specimen Type:	Whole blood precipitated with perchloric acid.
Reference:	Bonnefont JP, Specola NB, Vassault A, et al. The fasting test in paediatrics: application to the diagnosis of pathological hypo- and hyperketotic states. Eur J Pediatr; 1990;150:80-5.
Method(s):	Standard enzymatic procedure. See reference.
Comments:	The above results are 10 - 90th percentiles and refer to 15h fasting values. For 20 and 24h fasting values see reference.

5-HYDROXYINDOLEACETIC ACID (URINE)
(5HIAA)

Age	n	Male and Female		
		mg/24h	μmol/24h	mg/g creatinine
3 - 8y	76	0.4 - 5.6	2.1 - 29.3	1.2 - 16.2
9 - 12y	43	1.0 - 6.3	5.2 - 32.9	2.4 - 8.7
13 - 17y	43	0.9 - 6.5	4.7 - 34.0	1.8 - 5.5
Adults	51	1.0 - 7.0	5.2 - 36.6	1.3 - 6.9

Specimen Type:	Urine
Reference:	Nichols Institute. Pediatric Endocrine Testing 1993:24.
Method(s):	Fluorescent polarization.
Comments:	Results are 2.5 - 97.5th percentiles.

17a-HYDROXYPROGESTERONE
(17α-OHP)

Test	Age	n	ng/dL	nmol/L	n	ng/dL	nmol/L
		Male			**Female**		
1.	1 - 30d	45	53 - 186	1.6 - 5.6	51	17 - 204	0.5 - 6.2
	31 - 182d	48	35 - 157	1.1 - 4.8	46	25 - 110	0.8 - 3.3
	183 - 365d	27	6 - 40	0.2 - 1.2	34	5 - 47	0.2 - 1.4
	1 - 3y	104	2 - 19	0.1 - 0.6	77	3 - 51	0.1 - 1.5
	4 - 6y	91	1 - 34	0.0 - 1.0	64	4 - 34	0.1 - 1.0
	7 - 9y	74	1 - 45	0.0 - 1.4	53	4 - 44	0.1 - 1.3
	10 - 12y	89	1 - 34	0.0 - 1.0	45	3 - 33	0.1 - 1.0
	13 - 15y	61	23 - 82	0.7 - 2.5	42	2 - 72	0.1 - 2.2
	16 - 18y	33	8 - 100	0.2 - 3.0	38	3 - 91	0.1 - 2.8

Test	Age	n	ng/dL	nmol/L
			Male and Female	
2.	0 - 1d	*	170 - 2500	5 - 75
	1 - 7d	*	30 – 350	1 – 10
	7 - 28d	*	0 - 250	0 – 8
	1 – 12mo	*	0 – 170	0 – 5
	1 - <4y	*	0 - 100	0 – 3
	4 - <10y(P$_1$)	*	0 – 100	0 – 3
	P$_2$	*	0 - 130	0 – 4
	P$_3$	*	30 – 200	1 – 6
	P$_4$	*	30 – 230	1 – 7
	P$_5$	*	30 – 250	1 – 8

Specimen Type:	1, 2	Serum or Plasma
Reference:	1. 2.	Soldin SJ, Bailey J, Beatey J, et al. Pediatric reference ranges for 17α-hydroxy-progesterone. Clin Chem 1995;41:S92 (Abstract). Soldin SJ, Rifai N, Hicks JM, Eds. Biochemical Basis of Pediatric Disease 3rd Edition. AACC Press, 1998; Chapter 9 p. 233.
Method(s):	1. 2.	Coat-a-count (Diagnostic Products Corporation, Los Angeles, CA). See reference
Comments:	1. 2.	Study used hospitalized patients and a computerized approach adapted from the Hoffmann technique. Values are 2.5 - 97.5th percentiles. These reference ranges are for guidance only. Numbers not provided. P_1 – P_5 refers to pubertal stages.

IGF BINDING PROTEIN-3

	Age	n	Male and Female mg/L
1.	2 - 23mo	40	0.7 - 2.3
	2 - 7y	36	0.9 - 4.1
	8 - 11y	68	1.5 - 4.3
	12 – 18y	207	2.2 - 4.2
	19 – 55y	137	2.0 - 4.0
2.	0 - 1w	32	0.42 - 1.39
	1 - 4w	16	0.77 - 2.09
	1 - 3mo	20	0.87 - 2.54
	3 - 6mo	18	0.98 - 2.64
	6 - 12mo	25	1.07 - 2.76
	1 - 3y	36	1.41 - 2.97
	3 - 5y	22	1.52 - 3.32
	5 - 7y	25	1.66 - 3.59
	7 - 9y	47	1.82 - 3.80
	9 - 11y	50	2.12 - 4.26
	11 – 13y	77	2.22 - 4.89
	13 – 15y	77	2.31 - 5.24
	15 – 17y	42	2.33 - 4.95
	20 – 30y	32	2.20 - 4.93

Specimen Type:	1,2 Serum
Reference:	1. Nichols Institute. Pediatric Endocrine Testing, 1993;26. 2. Blum WF, Ranke MB, Kietzmann K, et al. A specific radio-immunoassay for the growth hormone (GH)-dependent somato-medin-binding protein: Its use for diagnosis of GH deficiency. J Clin Endocrinol Metab 1990;70:1292-8.
Method(s):	1,2 Radioimmunoassay
Comments:	1. Results are 2.5 - 97.5th percentiles. 2. Results are 5 - 95th percentiles.

IMMUNOGLOBULIN A
(IgA)

Test	Age	n	mg/dL	g/L
1.	0 – 12mo	75	0 - 100	0.00 - 1.00
	1 – 3y	52	24 - 121	0.24 - 1.21
	4 – 6y	41	33 - 235	0.33 - 2.35
	7 – 9y	55	41 - 368	0.41 - 3.68
	10 – 11y	38	64 - 246	0.64 - 2.46
	12 – 13y	38	70 - 432	0.70 - 4.32
	14 – 15y	38	57 - 300	0.57 - 3.00
	16 – 19y	74	0.74 - 4.19	0.74 - 4.19

Test	Age	Male			Female		
		n	mg/dL	g/L	n	mg/dL	g/L
2.	1 - 30d	61	1 - 20	0.01 - 0.20	56	1 - 19	0.01 - 0.19
	31 - 182d	52	7 - 56	0.07 - 0.56	60	1 - 59	0.01 - 0.59
	183 - 365d	37	9 - 107	0.09 - 1.07	23	15 - 90	0.15 - 0.90
	1 - 3y	105	18 - 171	0.18 - 1.71	127	25 - 141	0.25 - 1.41
	4 - 6y	138	60 - 231	0.60 - 2.31	135	47 - 206	0.47 - 2.06
	7 - 9y	111	77 - 252	0.77 - 2.52	105	41 - 218	0.41 - 2.18
	10 - 12y	104	61 - 269	0.61 - 2.69	115	73 - 239	0.73 - 2.39
	13 - 15y	104	42 - 304	0.42 - 3.04	118	82 - 296	0.82 - 2.96
	16 - 18y	112	89 - 314	0.89 - 3.14	100	90 - 322	0.90 - 3.22

Specimen Type:	1.	Plasma
	2.	Serum or plasma
Reference:	1.	Lockitch G, Halstead AC, Quigley G, et al. Age and sex specific pediatric reference intervals: Study design and methods illustrated by measurement of serum proteins with the Behring LN Nephelometer. Clin Chem 1988;34:1618-21.
	2.	Soldin SJ, Bailey J, Beatey J, et al. Pediatric reference ranges for immunoglobulins G, A and M on the Behring nephelometer. Clin Chem 1996;42:S308. (Abstract)
Method(s):	1,2	Nephelometry (Behring Diagnostics, Inc., Westwood MA).
Comments:	1.	Study performed on healthy normal children. Results are 2.5 - 97.5th percentiles.
	2.	Study used hospitalized patients and a computerized approach adapted from the Hoffmann technique to obtain the 2.5 - 97.5th percentiles.

112

IMMUNOGLOBULIN D (IgD)				
	Male and Female			
Age	n	mg/dL	n	mg/L
Newborn	*	None detected	*	None detected
Thereafter	*	0 - 8		0 - 80
Specimen Type:	Serum			
Reference:	Behrman RE, Ed. Nelson textbook of pediatrics, 14th ed. Philadelphia, PA: WB Saunders Company, 1992:1813.			
Method(s):	Not given.			
Comments:	*Numbers not provided in reference.			

IMMUNOGLOBULIN E
(IgE)

Test	Age	n	Male KIU/L	n	Female KIU/L
1.	0 - 12mo	40	2 - 24	29	0 - 20
	1 - 3y	74	2 - 149	104	2 - 55
	4 - 10y	155	4 - 249	124	8 - 279
	11 - 15y	137	7 - 280	152	5 - 295
	16 - 18y	58	5 - 268	67	7 - 698
2.	0 - 12mo	28	< 12	28	< 8
	1 - 3y	44	< 90	67	< 28
	4 - 10y	76	< 163	56	< 137
	11 - 18y	96	< 179	109	< 398

Specimen Type:	1,2	Serum, Plasma
Reference:	1.	Soldin SJ, Morales A, Albalos F, et al. Pediatric reference ranges on the Abbott IMx for FSH, LH, prolactin, TSH, T_4, T_3, free t_4, free T_3, T-uptake, IgE and ferritin. Clin Biochem 1995;28:603-6.
	2.	Soldin SJ, Lenherr S, Kumar A. Pediatric reference ranges for IgE. Clin Chem 1995;41:S92. (Abstract)
Method(s):	1.	Abbott IMx (Abbott Laboratories, Abbott Park, IL)
	2.	Behring LN Nephelometer (Behring Diagnostics, Westwood MA).
Comments:	1,2	Study performed on hospitalized patients and the Hoffmann technique applied to obtain the 2.5 - 97.5th percentiles (1) and 97.5th percentile (2).

IMMUNOGLOBULIN G
(IgG)

Test	Age	Male and Female		
		n	mg/dL	g/L
1.	0 - 12mo	75	273 - 1660	2.73 - 16.60
	1 - 3y	52	533 - 1078	5.33 - 10.78
	4 - 6y	41	593 - 1723	5.93 - 17.23
	7 - 9y	55	673 - 1734	6.73 - 17.34
	10 - 11y	38	821 - 1835	8.21 - 18.35
	12 - 13y	38	893 - 1823	8.93 - 18.23
	14 - 15y	38	842 - 2013	8.42 - 20.13
	16 - 19y	74	646 - 1864	6.46 - 18.64

Test	Age	Male			Female		
		n	mg/dL	g/L	n	mg/dL	g/L
2.	1 - 30d	61	260 - 986	2.60 - 9.86	56	221 - 1031	2.21 - 10.31
	31 - 182d	52	195 - 643	1.95 - 6.43	60	390 - 794	3.90 - 7.94
	183 - 365d	37	184 - 974	1.84 - 9.74	23	407 - 774	4.07 - 7.74
	1 - 3y	105	507 - 1305	5.07 - 13.05	127	550 - 1407	5.50 - 14.07
	4 - 6y	138	571 - 1550	5.71 - 15.50	135	675 - 1540	6.75 - 15.40
	7 - 9y	111	700 - 1680	7.00 - 16.80	105	589 - 1717	5.89 - 17.17
	10 - 12y	104	818 - 1885	8.18 - 18.85	115	705 - 1871	7.05 - 18.71
	13 - 15y	104	709 - 1861	7.09 - 18.61	118	891 - 1907	8.91 - 19.07
	16 - 18y	112	632 - 1979	6.32 - 19.79	100	953 - 2108	9.53 - 21.08

Specimen Type:
1. Plasma
2. Serum or plasma

Reference:

1. Lockitch G, Halstead AC, Quigley G, et al. Age and sex specific pediatric reference intervals: Study design and methods illustrated by measurement of serum proteins with the Behring LN Nephelometer. Clin Chem 1988;34:1618-21.

2. Soldin SJ, Bailey J, Beatey J, et al. Pediatric reference ranges for immunoglobulins G, A and M on the Behring nephelometer. Clin Chem 1996;42:S308. (Abstract)

Method(s):

1,2 Nephelometry (Behring Diagnostics, Inc., Westwood, MA).

Comments:

1. Study performed on healthy normal children.
Results are 2.5 - 97.5 percentiles.

2. Study used hospitalized patients and a computerized approach adapted from the Hoffmann technique to obtain the 2.5 - 97.5th percentiles.

IMMUNOGLOBULIN M
(IgM)

Test	Age	n	Male mg/dL	Male g/L	Female mg/dL	Female g/L
1.	0 - 12mo	75	0 - 216	0.00 - 2.16	0 - 216	0.00 - 2.16
	1 - 3y	52	28 - 218	0.28 - 2.18	28 - 218	0.28 - 2.18
	4 - 6y	41	36 - 314	0.36 - 3.14	36 - 314	0.36 - 3.14
	7 - 9y	55	47 - 311	0.47 - 3.11	47 - 311	0.47 - 3.11
	10 - 11y	38	46 - 268	0.46 - 2.68	46 - 268	0.46 - 2.68
	12 - 13y	38	52 - 357	0.52 - 3.57	52 - 357	0.52 - 3.57
	14 - 15y	38	23 - 281	0.23 - 2.81	23 - 281	0.23 - 2.81
	16 - 19y	74	35 - 387	0.35 - 3.87	35 - 387	0.35 - 3.87

Test	Age	n	Male mg/dL	Male g/L	n	Female mg/dL	Female g/L
2.	1 - 30d	61	12 - 117	0.12 - 1.17	56	19 - 104	0.19 - 1.04
	31 - 182d	52	27 - 147	0.27 - 1.47	60	9 - 212	0.09 - 2.12
	183 - 365d	37	41 - 197	0.41 - 1.97	23	4 - 216	0.04 - 2.16
	1 - 3y	105	63 - 240	0.63 - 2.40	127	70 - 298	0.70 - 2.98
	4 - 6y	138	64 - 248	0.64 - 2.48	135	81 - 298	0.81 - 2.98
	7 - 9y	111	49 - 231	0.49 - 2.31	105	62 - 270	0.62 - 2.70
	10 - 12y	104	58 - 249	0.58 - 2.49	115	81 - 340	0.81 - 3.40
	13 - 15y	104	57 - 298	0.57 - 2.98	118	69 - 361	0.69 - 3.61
	16 - 18y	112	59 - 291	0.59 - 2.91	100	86 - 360	0.86 - 3.60

Specimen Type:	1. Plasma 2. Serum or plasma
Reference:	1. Lockitch G, Halstead AC, Quigley G, et al. Age and sex specific pediatric reference intervals: Study design and methods illustrated by measurement of serum proteins with the Behring LN Nephelometer. Clin Chem 1988;34:1618-21. 2. Soldin SJ, Bailey J, Beatey J, et al. Pediatric reference ranges for immunoglobulins G, A and M on the Behring nephelometer. Clin Chem 1996;42:S308. (Abstract)
Method(s):	1,2 Nephelometry (Behring Diagnostics, Inc., Westwood MA).
Comments:	1. Study performed on healthy normal children. Results are 2.5 - 97.5th percentiles. 2. Study used hospitalized patients and a computerized approach adapted from the Hoffmann technique to obtain the 2.5 - 97.5th percentiles.

IMMUNOGLOBULIN LIGHT CHAINS
(KAPPA AND LAMBDA)

Age	n	Kappa mg/dL	Kappa g/L	Lambda mg/dL	Lambda g/L
Newborn	325	770 - 870	7.7 - 8.7	170 - 190	1.7 - 1.9
Premature	168	310 - 490	3.1 - 4.9	160 - 190	1.6 - 1.9
1mo	50	360 - 480	3.6 - 4.8	160 - 200	1.6 - 2.0
2mo	50	240 - 270	2.4 - 2.7	160 - 170	1.6 - 1.7
3mo	50	170 - 250	1.7 - 2.5	100 - 130	1.0 - 1.3
4mo	50	190 - 240	1.9 - 2.4	80 - 100	0.8 - 1.0
5mo	50	200 - 320	2.0 - 3.2	100 - 110	1.0 - 1.1
1y	50	300 - 530	3.0 - 5.3	90 - 120	0.9 - 1.2
2y	50	360 - 640	3.6 - 6.4	130 - 150	1.3 - 1.5
3y	50	410 - 540	4.1 - 5.4	110 - 140	1.1 - 1.4
4y	50	480 - 830	4.8 - 8.3	120 - 170	1.2 - 1.7
5y	50	540 - 710	5.4 - 7.1	130 - 170	1.3 - 1.7
6y	50	600 - 850	6.0 - 8.5	160 - 170	1.6 - 1.7
7y	50	460 - 750	4.6 - 7.5	140 - 180	1.4 - 1.8
8y	50	730 - 910	7.3 - 9.1	140 - 170	1.4 - 1.7
9y	50	710 - 960	7.1 - 9.6	150 - 180	1.5 - 1.8
10y	50	820 - 960	8.2 - 9.6	130 - 190	1.3 - 1.9
11y	50	600 - 830	6.0 - 8.3	140 - 180	1.4 - 1.8
12y	50	820 - 960	8.2 - 9.6	170 - 200	1.7 - 2.0
13y	50	820 - 1050	8.2 - 10.5	140 - 170	1.4 - 1.7
14y	50	800 - 1080	8.0 - 10.8	190 - 220	1.9 - 2.2
15y	50	720 - 1100	7.2 - 11.0	170 - 230	1.7 - 2.3
16y	50	700 - 1120	7.0 - 11.2	150 - 220	1.5 - 2.2

Specimen Type:	Serum
Reference:	Herkner KR, Salzer H, Böck A, et al. Pediatric and perinatal reference intervals for immunoglobulin light chains kappa and lambda. Clin Chem 1992;38:548-50.
Method(s):	Nephelometry. Kallestad Model CPM 300 (Diagnostics Pasteur, Marnes-la-Coquette, France).
Comments:	The subjects were healthy newborns and children who had been screened to rule out immunological disorders and infections. The ranges are 10 - 90th percentiles.

IMMUNOGLOBULIN G SUBCLASS
(IgG - SUBCLASS)

Age	n	Male and Female, g/L (To convert to mg/dL, multiply by 100)			
		IgG$_1$	IgG$_2$	IgG$_3$	IgG$_4$
Cord Blood Serum Preterm	20	3.4 - 9.7	0.7 - 1.7	0.2 - 0.5	0.2 - 0.7
Cord Blood Serum Term	20	5.8 - 13.7	0.6 - 5.2	0.2 - 1.2	0.2 - 1.0
5y	20	5.6 - 12.7	0.4 - 4.4	0.3 - 1.0	0.1 - 0.8
6y	20	6.2 - 11.3	0.5 - 4.0	0.3 - 0.8	0.2 - 0.9
7y	20	5.4 - 10.5	0.9 - 3.5	0.3 - 1.1	0.2 - 1.1
8y	20	5.6 - 10.5	0.7 - 4.5	0.2 - 1.1	0.1 - 0.8
9y	20	3.9 - 11.4	0.7 - 4.7	0.4 - 1.2	0.2 - 1.0
10y	20	4.4 - 10.8	0.6 - 4.0	0.3 - 1.2	0.1 - 0.9
11y	20	6.4 - 10.9	0.9 - 4.3	0.3 - 0.9	0.2 - 1.0
12y	20	6.0 - 11.5	0.9 - 4.8	0.4 - 1.0	0.2 - 0.9
13y	20	6.1 - 11.5	0.9 - 7.9	0.2 - 1.1	0.1 - 0.8
Adults	20	4.8 - 9.5	1.1 - 6.9	0.3 - 0.8	0.2 - 1.1

Specimen Type:	Serum
Reference:	Miles J, Riches P. The determination of IgG subclass concentrations in serum by enzyme linked immunosorbent assay: establishment of age-related reference ranges for cord blood samples, children aged 5-13 years and adults. Ann Clin Biochem 1994;31:24-8.
Method(s):	ELISA
Comments:	Cord blood samples were obtained from both premature and term infants. Samples were obtained from school children and adults. Results are 5 - 95th percentiles.

INSULIN-LIKE GROWTH FACTOR-1 (IGF-1)
SOMATOMEDIN-C

Test	Age	Male			Female		
		n	nmol/L	ng/mL	n	nmol/L	ng/mL
1.	1 - 30d	34	0.2 - 7.3	2 - 56	31	0.9 - 11.9	7 - 92
	31 - 182d	55	0.2 - 10.6	2 - 82	61	0.6 - 9.4	5 - 72
	183 - 365d	27	0.2 - 7.0	2 - 54	35	1.1 - 9.8	8 - 75
	1 - 3y	140	2.2 - 15.0	17 - 116	111	1.6 - 17.5	12 - 135
	4 - 6y	126	2.7 - 20.8	21 - 160	83	1.7 - 22.8	13 - 176
	7 - 9y	100	8.4 - 26.9	65 - 207	74	6.9 - 32.9	53 - 253
	10 - 12y	113	9.0 - 25.4	69 - 196	86	9.8 - 46.3	75 - 357
	13 - 15y	116	10.4 - 52.5	80 - 404	94	8.6 - 44.7	66 - 344
	16 - 18y	62	12.5 - 49.7	96 - 383	85	12.8 - 47.3	99 - 364
2.	2mo - 5y	97	2.2 - 32.2	17 - 248	97	2.2 - 32.2	17 - 248
	6 - 8y	40	11.4 - 61.5	88 - 474	40	11.4 - 61.5	88 - 474
	9 - 11y	125	14.2 - 73.4	110 - 565	174	15.2 - 100.1	117 - 771
	12 - 15y	135	26.2 - 124.3	202 - 957	195	33.9 - 142.3	261 - 1096
	16 - 24y	95	23.6 - 101.3	182 - 780	95	23.6 - 101.3	182 - 780

Specimen Type:	1,2 Serum
Reference:	1. Soldin SJ, Hicks JM, Bailey J, et al. Pediatric reference ranges for creatine kinase and insulin-like growth factor 1. Clin Chem 1997;43:S199. (Abstract) 2. Nichols Institute Test Catalogue, 1996.
Method(s):	1. Radioimmunoassay, IncStar® (IncStar Corporation, Stillwater, MN) 2. Radioimmunoassay
Comments:	1. Results are 2.5 - 95th percentiles. Study used hospitalized patients and a computerized adaptation of the Hoffmann technique. 2. Results are 2.5 - 97.5th percentiles.

INSULIN-LIKE GROWTH FACTOR – II (IGF – II)

Test	Age	Males		Females	
		n	ng/mL μg/L	n	ng/mL μg/L
1.	<3y	10	310 - 650	10	129 – 709
	3 – 5y	9	55 - 1091	15	124 - 928
	6 - 8y	15	237 - 977	20	145 - 1057
	9 – 11y	10	127 - 883	16	252 - 792
	12 – 14y	38	272 – 728	26	266 - 730
	>15y	14	317 - 745	14	176 - 756

Specimen Type:	1	Plasma
Reference:	1.	Rosenfeld RG, Wilson DM, Lee PDK, et al. Insulin-like growth factors I and II in evaluation of growth retardation., J Ped 1986; 109:428-33
Method(s):	1.	RIA after gel filtration on Sephadex G-50. See reference above.
Comments:	1.	Subjects were normal healthy children, with heights between the 5th and 95th percentiles for age, selected from an outpatient pediatric clinic. Results are 2.5 – 97.5[th] percentiles.

		Male			Female		
IRON								
Test	**Age**	**n**	**µg/dL**	**µmol/L**	**n**	**µg/dL**	**µmol/L**
1.	1 - 5y*	44*	22 - 136	4 - 25	44*	22 - 136	4 - 25
	6 - 9y*	50*	39 - 136	7 - 25	50*	39 - 136	7 - 25
	10 - 14y	31	28 - 134	5 - 24	40	45 - 145	8 - 26
	14 - 19y	65	34 - 162	6 - 29	110	28 - 184	5 - 33
2.	1 - 30d	80	32 - 112	5.7 - 20.0	44	29 - 127	5.2 - 22.7
	31 - 365d	87	27 - 109	4.8 - 19.5	75	25 - 126	4.5 - 22.6
	1 - 3y	160	29 - 91	5.2 - 16.3	119	25 - 101	4.5 - 18.1
	4 - 6y	114	25 - 115	4.5 - 20.6	88	28 - 93	5.0 - 16.7
	7 - 9y	116	27 - 96	4.8 - 17.2	101	30 - 104	5.4 - 18.6
	10 - 12y	107	28 - 112	5.0 - 20.0	91	32 - 104	5.7 - 18.6
	13 - 15y	98	26 - 110	4.7 - 19.7	117	30 - 109	5.4 - 19.5
	16 - 18y	92	27 - 138	4.8 - 24.7	99	33 - 102	5.9 - 18.3

		Male and Female					
3.		**5 – 11am**			**5 – 11pm**		
	Age	**n**	**µg/dL**	**µmol/L**	**n**	**µg/dL**	**µmol/L**
	0 – 24mo	332	20 – 105	3.6 – 18.8	43	20 – 140	3.6 – 25.0
	2 – 9y	370	20 – 105	3.6 – 18.8	100	20 – 145	3.6 – 26.0
	10 – 14y	145	20 – 100	3.6 – 17.9	43	20 – 145	3.6 – 26.0
	15 – 18y	125	20 – 100	3.6 – 17.9	42	20 - 145	3.6 – 26.0

Specimen Type:	1.	Plasma
	2, 3.	Plasma, Serum

Reference:	1.	Lockitch G, Halstead A, Wadsworth L, et al. Age and sex specific pediatric reference intervals for zinc, copper, selenium, iron, vitamins A and E and related proteins. Clin Chem 1988;34:1625-8.
	2.	Soldin SJ, Bailey J, Bjorn J, et al. Pediatric reference ranges for iron on the Hitachi 747 with Boehringer Mannheim reagents. Clin Chem 1999;45:A22. (Abstract)
	3.	Soldin SJ, Murthy JN, Agarwalla Pk, et al. Pediatric Reference Ranges for Creatine Kinase, CKMB, Troponin I, Iron and Cortisol. Clin Biochem 1999;32:77-80.

Method(s):	1.	Ferrozine (Sigma Chemical Company). RA-100 Analyzer, Technicon Instruments, Tarrytown, NY.
	2.	Hitachi 747 with Boehringer Mannheim reagents (Boehringer Mannheim Diagnostics, Indianapolis, IN)
	3.	Vitros 500 analyzer using Vitros reagents (Johnson and Johnson, Rochester, NY)

Comments:	1.	The study population was healthy children. Non-parametric methods were used to determine the 0.025 and 0.975 fractiles.
	2, 3.	Study used hospitalized patients and a computerized approach adapted from the Hoffmann technique. Values are the 2.5 - 97.5th percentiles. Results are somewhat lower than expected and represent data from a largely inner city population.

*No significant differences were found for males and females.
These ranges were therefore derived from combined data.

IRON BINDING CAPACITY, TOTAL (TIBC)

Test	Age	Male			Female		
		n	µg/dL	µmol/L	n	µg/dL	µmol/L
1.	1 - 5y*	44	268 - 441	48 - 79	44	268 - 441	48 - 79
	6 - 9y*	50	240 - 508	43 - 91	50	240 - 508	43 - 91
	10 - 14y	31	302 - 508	54 - 91	40	318 - 575	57 - 103
	14 - 19y	65	290 - 570	52 - 102	110	302 - 564	52 - 101
2.	1 - 30d	133	94 - 232	16.8 - 41.5	57	94 - 236	16.8 - 42.2
	31 - 182d	78	116 - 322	20.8 - 57.6	69	89 - 311	15.9 - 55.7
	183 - 365d	39	176 - 384	31.5 - 68.7	27	138 - 365	24.7 - 65.3
	1 - 3y	131	204 - 382	36.5 - 68.3	103	184 - 377	32.9 - 67.5
	4 - 6y	114	180 - 390	32.2 - 69.8	107	162 - 352	29.0 - 63.0
	7 - 9y	116	183 - 369	32.8 - 66.1	113	167 - 336	29.9 - 60.1
	10 - 12y	104	173 - 356	31.0 - 63.7	112	198 - 383	35.4 - 68.6
	13 - 15y	106	193 - 377	34.5 - 67.5	143	169 - 358	30.3 - 64.1
	16 - 18y	113	174 - 351	31.1 - 62.8	137	194 - 372	34.7 - 66.6

Specimen Type:	1.	Plasma
	2.	Serum
Reference:	1.	Lockitch G, Halstead A, Wadsworth L, et al. Age and sex specific pediatric reference intervals for zinc, copper, selenium, iron, vitamins A and E and related proteins. Clin Chem 1988;34:1625-8.
	2.	Soldin SJ, Hicks JM, Bailey J, et al. Pediatric reference ranges for total iron binding capacity and transferrin. Clin Chem 1997;43:S200. (Abstract)
Method(s):	1.	Transferrin was measured by nephelometry. Behring LN with Behring kit (Behringwerke, Marburg, Germany). Calculated TIBC.
	2.	Hitachi 747 using Boehringer-Mannheim reagents (Boehringer-Mannheim Diagnostics, Indianapolis, IN).
Comments:	1.	Values are 2.5 - 97.5th percentiles. Transferrin iron-binding capacity calculated by multiplying the transferrin g/L x 23.1.
		*No significant differences were found for males and females. These ranges were therefore derived from combined data.
	2.	Study used hospitalized patients and a computerized approach adapted from the Hoffmann technique. Values are 2.5 - 97.5th percentiles.

LACTATE

Test	Age	Male and Female		
		n	mg/dL	mmol/L
1.	1 - 12mo	12	10 - 21	1.1 - 2.3
	1 - 7y	27	7 - 14	0.8 - 1.5
	7 - 15y	9	5 - 8	0.6 - 0.9
2.	All ages	*	6.3 - 18.9	0.7 - 2.1

Specimen Type:	1. Whole blood precipitated with perchloric acid. 2. Plasma
Reference:	1. Bonnefont JP, Specola NB, Vassault A, et al. The fasting test in pediatrics: application to pathological hypo- and hyperketotic states. Eur J Pediatr 1990;150:80-5. 2. Children's National Medical Center. Unpublished data.
Method(s):	1. Standard enzymatic procedure. See reference. 2. Kodak Ektachem 500 (Johnson & Johnson, Rochester, NY).
Comments:	1. The above results are 10 - 90th percentiles and refer to 15h fasting values. For 20 and 24h fasting values, see reference. 2. *Numbers not available.

LACTATE DEHYDROGENASE
(LDH)

Test	Age	Male n	Male U/L	Female n	Female U/L
1.	1 - 30d	119	550 - 2100	76	580 – 2000
	1 - 3mo	108	480 - 1220	84	460 – 1150
	4 - 6mo	100	400 - 1230	54	480 – 1150
	7 - 12mo	97	380 - 1200	75	460 – 1060
2.	1 - 3y	50*	500 - 920	50*	500 – 920
	4 - 6y	40*	470 - 900	40*	470 – 900
	7 - 9y	80*	420 - 750	80*	420 – 750
	10 - 11y	27	432 - 700	34	380 – 700
	12 - 13y	31	470 - 750	49	380 – 640
	14 - 15y	26	360 - 730	52	390 – 580
	16 - 19y	40	340 - 670	61	340 – 670
3.	1 - 30d	77	125 - 735	65	145 – 765
	31 - 365d	86	170 - 450	74	190 – 420
	1 - 3y	135	155 - 345	109	165 – 395
	4 - 6y	101	155 - 345	96	135 – 345
	7 - 9y	125	145 - 300	104	140 – 280
	10 - 12y	111	120 - 325	76	120 – 260
	13 - 15y	105	120 - 290	101	100 – 275
	16 - 18y	79	105 - 235	98	105 – 230

Specimen Type:
1. Serum or Plasma
2, 3 Plasma

Reference:

1. Soldin SJ, Savwoir TV, Guo Y. Pediatric reference ranges for lactate dehydrogenase and uric acid during the first year of life on the Vitros 500 analyzer. Clin Chem 1997;43:S199. (Abstract)

2. Lockitch G, Halstead AC, Albersheim S, et al. Age and sex specific pediatric reference intervals for biochemistry analytes as measured with the Ektachem 700 analyzer. Clin Chem 1988;34:1622-5.

3. Soldin SJ, Bailey J, Bjorn S, et al. Pediatric reference ranges for LDH. Clin Chem 1995;41:S93. (Abstract)

Method(s):

1, 2 Ektachem 500 (1) and 700 (2) (Johnson & Johnson, Rochester, NY).

3. Measured on the Hitachi 747 using Boehringer-Mannheim reagents. (Boehringer-Mannheim Diagnostics, Indianapolis, IN.)

Comments:

1, 3 Study used hospitalized patients and a computerized approach adapted from the Hoffmann technique to obtain the 2.5 - 97.5th percentiles.

2. The study population was healthy children. Non-parametric methods were used to determine the 0.025 and 0.975 fractiles.

*No significant differences were found for males and females.
These ranges were therefore derived from combined data.

LACTATE/PYRUVATE RATIO

Age	n	Male and Female	
		Fed	15h Fast
1mo - 1y	12	--	10 - 28
1 - 7y	27	12 - 18	11 - 18
7 - 15y	9	8 - 20	8 - 20

Specimen Type:	See Lactate and Pyruvate.
Reference:	Hommes FA, Ed. Techniques in diagnostic human biochemical genetics. New York, NY: Wiley-Liss 1991:300.
Method(s):	See references for lactate and pyruvate.
Comments:	Results are 10 - 90th percentiles.

LEAD			
		Male and Female	
Age	**n**	**µg/dL**	**µmol/L**
0 - 15y	*	< 10	< 0.48

Specimen Type:	Whole blood.
Reference:	University of Virginia Health Sciences Center. Laboratory Medicine Update, Vol. 7, No. 24, May 9, 1994, pp. 3-4, and Children's National Medical Center, Washington, DC.
Method(s):	Atomic Absorption.
Comments:	CDC guidelines places the threshold for concern at 10 µg/dL. Results > 15 µg/dL are reported to Health Department for follow-up. *Numbers not provided.

LIPASE

Test	Age	Male and Female	
		n	U/L
1.	1 - 30d	83	6 - 55
	31 - 182d	121	4 - 29
	183 - 365d	56	4 - 23
	1 - 3y	148	4 - 31
	4 - 9y	96	3 - 32
	10 - 18y	142	4 - 29

	Age	Male		Female	
2.		n	U/L	n	U/L
	0- 90d	39*	10 - 85	39*	10 - 85
	3 – 12mo	113	13 - 95	137	9 - 128
	1 - <2y	118	15 - 135	222	15 - 150
	2 - <7y	323	15 – 175	243	10 - 150
	7 - <11y	216	10 – 175	209	13 - 150
	11 - <15y	75	10 – 195	150	10 - 180
	15 - 18y	70	10 – 195	79	10 - 220

Specimen Type: 1, 2 Plasma, Serum

Reference:
1. Soldin SJ, Bailey J., Beatey J., et al. Pediatric reference ranges for Lipase. Clin Chem 1995; 41:S93 (Abstract).

2. Soldin SJ, Ojeifo O. Pediatric reference ranges for lipase. Clin Chem 1999;45:A22. (Abstract)

Method(s):
1. Hitachi 717 using Sigma reagents (Boehringer-Mannheim Diagnostics, Indianapolis, IN).
2. Vitros 500 using Vitros reagents (Johnson & Johnson, Rochester, NY).

Comments: 1,2. Study used hospitalized patients and a computerized approach to removing outliers. Values are 2.5 - 97.5th percentiles.

LOW-DENSITY LIPOPROTEIN-CHOLESTEROL (LDL-C)

Test	Age	Male and Female		
		n	mmol/L	mg/dL
1.	2 – 12mo	100	0.82 - 3.02	32 - 117
	2 – 10y	120	0.98 - 3.62	38 - 140

2.		Male			Female		
		n	mmol/L	mg/dL	n	mmol/L	mg/dL
	5 – 9y	*	1.63 – 3.34	63 – 129	*	1.76 – 3.63	68 – 140
	10 – 14y	*	1.66 – 3.44	64 - 133	*	1.76 – 3.52	68 – 136
	15 – 19y	*	1.61 – 3.37	62 - 130	*	1.53 – 3.55	59 - 137

Specimen Type: 1,2. Serum

Reference:
1. Baroni S, Scribano D, Valentini P, et al. Serum apolipoprotein A1, B, CII, CIII, E, and lipoprotein (a) levels in children. Clin Biochem 1996;29:603-5.
2. Soldin SJ, Rifai N, Hicks JM, Eds. Biochemical Basis of Pediatric Diesease 3rd Edition. AACC Press, 1998; Chapter 18, p.468.

Method(s):
1. Calculated as described in Friedewald WT, Levy RI, Frederickson DC. Estimation of the concentration of low density lipoprotein cholesterol in plasma, without use of the preparative ultracentrifuge. Clin Chem 1972;18:499-502.
2. See reference.

Comments:
1. Results are the 2.5 - 97.5th percentiles for healthy children.
2. Numbers of participants not provided. Results are 5 – 95th percentiles.

LUTEINIZING HORMONE
(LH)

Test	Age	Male n	Male U/L	Female n	Female U/L
1.	< 2y	179	0.5 - 1.9	33	< 0.5
	2 - 5y	138	< 0.5	94	< 0.5
	6 - 10y	96	< 0.5	136	< 0.5
	11 - 20y	89	0.5 - 5.3	263	0.5 - 9.0
2.	< 2y	179	1.3 - 2.8	33	< 1.3
	2 - 5y	138	< 1.3	94	< 1.3
	6 - 10y	96	< 1.3	136	< 1.3
	11 - 20y	89	1.3 - 5.7	263	1.3 - 10.2

Specimen Type:	1,2 Plasma, Serum
Reference:	1. Soldin SJ, Morales A, Albalos F, et al. Pediatric reference ranges on the Abbott IMx for FSH, LH, prolactin, TSH, T_4, T_3, free T_4, free T_3, T-uptake, IgE and ferritin. Clin Biochem 1995;28:603-6.
	2. Murthy JN, Hicks JM, Soldin SJ. Evaluation of the Technicon Immuno I Random Access Immunoassay Analyzer and calculation of pediatric reference ranges for endocrine tests, T-uptake and ferritin. Clin Biochem 1995;28:181-5.
Method(s):	1. IMx (Abbott Laboratories, Abbott, Park, IL).
	2. Immuno I (Bayer Corp., Tarrytown, NY).
Comments:	1,2 Study used hospitalized patients and a computerized approach to removing outliers. Values are 2.5 - 97.5th percentiles.

130

MAGNESIUM

Test	Age	Male			Female		
		n	mg/dL	mmol/L	n	mg/dL	mmol/L
1.	1 - 30d	68	1.7 - 2.4	0.70 - 0.99	18	1.7 - 2.5	0.70 - 1.03
	31 - 365d	62	1.6 - 2.5	0.66 - 1.03	37	1.9 - 2.4	0.78 - 0.99
	1 - 3y	140	1.7 - 2.4	0.70 - 0.99	103	1.7 - 2.4	0.70 - 0.99
	4 - 6y	120	1.7 - 2.4	0.70 - 0.99	63	1.7 - 2.2	0.70 - 0.91
	7 - 9y	118	1.7 - 2.3	0.70 - 0.95	102	1.6 - 2.3	0.66 - 0.95
	10 - 12y	111	1.6 - 2.2	0.66 - 0.91	74	1.6 - 2.2	0.66 - 0.91
	13 - 15y	84	1.6 - 2.3	0.66 - 0.95	113	1.6 - 2.3	0.66 - 0.95
	16 - 18y	73	1.5 - 2.2	0.62 - 0.91	92	1.5 - 2.2	0.62 - 0.91
2.	Premature 0 - 6d	48	1.6 - 2.7	0.65 - 1.10	48	1.6 - 2.7	0.65 - 1.10
	Newborns 0 - 6d	134	1.2 - 2.6	0.48 - 1.05	134	1.2 - 2.6	0.48 - 1.05
	Premature 7 - 30d	24	1.8 - 2.4	0.75 - 1.00	24	1.8 - 2.4	0.75 - 1.00
	Newborn 7 - 30d	89	1.6 - 2.4	0.65 - 1.00	89	1.6 - 2.4	0.65 - 1.00
	1m - 1y	164	1.6 - 2.6	0.65 - 1.05	164	1.6 - 2.6	0.65 - 1.05
	1 - 2y	102	1.6 - 2.6	0.65 - 1.05	102	1.6 - 2.6	0.65 - 1.05
	2 - 6y	138	1.5 - 2.4	0.60 - 1.00	138	1.5 - 2.4	0.60 - 1.00
	6 - 10y	130	1.6 - 2.3	0.65 - 0.95	130	1.6 - 2.3	0.65 - 0.95
	10 - 14y	133	1.6 - 2.2	0.65 - 0.90	133	1.6 - 2.2	0.65 - 0.90
	14y +	139	1.5 - 2.3	0.60 - 0.95	139	1.5 - 2.3	0.60 - 0.95

Specimen Type:	1, 2	Plasma
Reference:	1.	Hicks JM, Bailey J, Bjorn S, et al. Pediatric reference ranges for plasma magnesium. Clin Chem 1995;41:S93. (Abstract)
	2.	Meites S, Ed. Pediatric clinical chemistry, 3rd ed. Washington, DC: AACC Press, 1989:191.
Method(s):	1.	Magnesium reacts with calmagite to form a reddish violet chromophore. Hitachi 747 with Boehringer-Mannheim reagents. (Boehringer-Mannheim Diagnostics, Indianapolis, IN.)
	2.	Colorimetric using a formazan dye. Kodak Ektachem 700 (Johnson & Johnson, Rochester, NY).
Comments:	1.	Study used hospitalized patients and a computerized approach adapted from the Hoffmann technique to obtain 2.5 - 97.5th percentiles.
	2.	Results are 5 - 95th percentiles from patients at Children's Hospital, Columbus, OH. Males and females studied together.

Manganese

Age	n	Male and Female	
		µg/L	nmol/L
0 - <0.5y	13	0.5 – 3.8	8.7 – 68.7
0.5 - <1.0y	18	0.6 – 3.7	10.7 – 66.3
1.0 - <2.0y	15	0.0 – 3.4	0.0 – 61.1
2.0 - <4.0y	23	0.4 – 2.3	8.1 – 42.1
4.0 - <6.0y	19	0.2 – 2.7	3.3 – 49.3
6.0 - <10.0y	25	0.3 – 2.3	5.2 – 40.8
10.0 - <14.0y	21	0.4 – 2.0	7.6 – 36.4
14.0 - <18.0y	17	0.4 – 1.5	7.8 – 27.8

Specimen Type:	Serum/Plasma
Reference:	Rükgauer M, Klein J, Kruse – James JD. Reference Values for theTrace Elements Copper, Manganese, Selenium, and Zinc in the Serum/Plasma of Children, Adolescents, and Adults. J Trace Elements Med Biol 1997;11:92-8
Method(s):	Atomic Absorption Spectrophotometry with Zeeman background compensation. Perkin Elased ETAAS, Zeeman 3030, Uberlingen, Germany
Comments:	Study population was drawn from patients visiting the outpatient department or surgical or orthapedic ward for preoperative workup. Results are mean ± 2 SD s. (2.5th – 97.5th percentiles)

METANEPHRINE (URINE)

Age	n	Male and Female		
		µg/24h	µmol/24h	µg/g creatinine
3 - 8y	76	5 - 113	0.025 - 0.514	47 - 240
9 - 12y	44	21 - 154	0.107 - 0.782	40 - 220
13 - 17y	43	32 - 167	0.162 - 0.848	33 - 145
Adults	51	45 - 290	0.228 - 1.472	31 - 140

Specimen Type:	Urine
Reference:	Nichols Institute. Pediatric Endocrine Testing, 1993, p. 30.
Method(s):	HPLC electrochemical detection.
Comments:	Results are 2.5 - 97.5th percentiles.

METHYLMALONIC ACID

Age	n	Male and Female
		µmol/L
4 - 8y	19	0.06 - 0.24
8 - 14y	20	0. 03 - 0.26

Specimen Type:	Serum
Reference:	Straczek J, Felden F, Dousset B. Quantification of methylmalonic acid in serum measured by capillary gas chromatography-mass spectrometry as tert-butyldimethylsilyl derivates. J Chromat 1993:620;1-7.
Method(s):	Gas chromatography-mass spectrometry.
Comments:	Results are 2.5 - 97.5th percentiles.

β2-MICROGLOBULIN

Age	Male		Female	
	n	μg/L	n	μg/L
1 - 30d	68	1603 - 4790	50	1722 - 4547
31 - 182d	73	1423 - 3324	68	1024 - 3774
183 - 365d	39	897 - 3095	27	999 - 2282
1 - 3y	158	827 - 2228	129	742 - 2396
4 - 6y	142	567 - 2260	123	546 - 2170
7 - 9y	97	772 - 1712	79	736 - 1766
10 - 12y	92	699 - 1836	68	704 - 1951
13 - 15y	103	681 - 1954	82	787 - 1916
16 - 18y	54	724 - 1874	77	555 - 1852

Specimen Type:	Serum, Plasma
Reference:	Soldin SJ, Hicks JM, Bailey J, et al. Pediatric reference ranges for β2-microglobulin and ceruloplasmin. Clin Chem 1997;43:S199. (Abstract)
Method(s):	RIA. Pharmacia β2-Micro RIA (Pharmacia, Uppsala, Sweden)
Comments:	Study used hospitalized patients and a computerized approach adapted from the Hoffmann technique. Values are the 2.5 - 97.5th percentiles.

MUCOPOLYSACCHARIDES (URINE)

Age	n	Male and Female mg/mmol creatinine
0 - <6mo	102	15.2 – 52.0
6mo - <12mo	34	15.1 – 31.5
1 - <2y	43	9.1 – 29.9
2 - <4y	55	7.7 – 21.3
4 - <6y	45	7.6 – 14.4
6 - <8y	30	5.7 – 12.9
8 - <10y	16	5.2 – 11.6
10 - <15y	27	2.4 – 10.6
15 - <20y	10	1.5 – 6.7
>20y	31	1.5 – 5.1

Specimen Type:	Urine
Reference:	de Jong JGN, Wevers RA, Liebrand – van Sambeek R. Measuring Urinary Glycosaminoglycans in the Presence of Protein: An Improved Screening Procedure for Mucopolysaccharides Based on Dimethyl-methylene Blue. Clin Chem 1992; 36:803-7
Method(s):	Dimethylene blue – Tris assay
Comments:	Results are the 2.5 – 97.5th percentiles

NOREPINEPHRINE/NORADRENALINE
(PLASMA)

Test	Age	n	nmol/L	pg/mL
			Male and Female	
1.	2 - 10d	21	1.0 - 7.0	169 - 1184
	10d - 3mo	10	2.2 - 12.3	372 - 2081
	3mo - 1y	14	1.6 - 6.6	271 - 1117
	1 - 2y	13	0.4 - 10.7	68 - 1810
	2 - 3y	8	1.1 - 8.7	186 - 1472
	3 - 15y	20	0.5 - 7.4	85 - 1252
2.	30 min after birth	16	2.5 - 9.1	422 - 1538
	2 hours after birth	16	3.1 - 6.5	532 - 1108
	3 hours after birth	16	0.7 - 8.5	112 - 1436
	12 hours after birth	16	1.2 - 1.9	195 - 327
	24 hours after birth	16	1.5 - 2.8	250 - 470
	48 hours after birth	16	1.3 - 2.0	221 - 345

Specimen Type:	1,2 Plasma
Reference:	1. Candito M, Albertini M, Politano S, et al. Plasma catecholamine levels in children. J Chrom Biomed Appl 1993;617:304-7.
	2. Eliot RJ, Lam R, Leake RD, et al. Plasma catecholamine concentrations in infants at birth and during the first 48 hours of life. J Pediatrics 1980;96:311-5.
Method(s):	1. High performance liquid chromatography.
	2. Radioenzymatic method.
Comments:	1. Study population consisted of 86 healthy children (62 males, 24 females) aged 2 days to 15 years.
	2. Study performed on 16 term vaginally delivered infants. Results are mean ± 2SD.

NOREPINEPHRINE/NORADRENALINE
(URINE)

Test	Age	n	Male and Female	
			µg/g creatinine	mmol/mol creatinine
1.	0 - 24mo	24	< 420	< 0.280
	2 - 4y	37	< 120	< 0.080
	5 - 9y	40	< 89	< 0.059
	10 - 19y	41	< 82	< 0.055
2.	< 1y	18	25 - 310	0.017 - 0.207
	1 - 4y	24	25 - 290	0.017 - 0.194
	4 - 10y	23	27 - 108	0.018 - 0.072
	10 - 18y	20	4 - 105	0.003 – 0.070

Specimen Type:	1,2	Urine
Reference:	1.	Soldin SJ, Lam G, Pollard A, et al. High performance liquid chromatographic analysis of urinary catecholamines employing amperometric detection: Reference values and use in laboratory diagnosis of neural crest tumors. Clin Biochem 1980;13:285-91.
	2.	Rosano TG. Liquid chromatographic evaluation of age related changes in the urinary excretion of free catecholamines in pediatric patients. Clin Chem 1984;30:301-3.
Method(s):	1,2	HPLC with electrochemical detection.
Comments:	1.	Study involved healthy children. Results quoted are 95th percentile.
	2.	Urine was obtained from 85 pediatric patients (diagnosis of neoplasia excluded). Results are 0 - 100th percentiles.

NORMETANEPHRINE (URINE)

Age	n	Male and Female		
		µg/24h	µmol/24h	µg/g creatinine
3 - 8y	76	13 - 252	0.071 - 1.375	62 - 705
9 - 12y	44	32 - 346	0.175 - 1.888	81 - 583
13 - 17y	43	63 - 402	0.344 - 2.194	95 - 375
Adults	51	82 - 500	0.448 - 2.729	47 - 310

Specimen Type:	Urine
Reference:	Nichols Institute. Pediatric Endocrine Testing, 1993, p. 30.
Method(s):	HPLC electrochemical detection.
Comments:	Results are 2.5 - 97.5th percentiles.

OSMOLALITY

Test	Age	Male and Female	
		n	mOsm/Kg
1.	Birth	44	275 - 300
	7d	17	276 - 305
	28d	17	274 - 305
2.	Adults	*	282 - 300

Specimen Type:	1,2 Serum
Reference:	1. Davies DP. Plasma osmolality and protein intake in preterm infants. Arch Dis Child 1973;48:575-9. Meites S, Ed. Pediatric Clinical Chemistry, 3rd ed. Washington, DC: AACC Press, 1989:202-3. 2. Pesce AJ, Kaplan LA. Methods in clinical chemistry. Washington DC: CV Mosby Co., 1987:20.
Method(s):	Freezing-point depression
Comments:	1. The report is based on Davies' study of 53 preterm infants with birthweights < 2.5 Kg. 2. *Number not provided.

OXYGEN, PARTIAL PRESSURE
(pO₂)

Age	n	Male and Female	
		mm Hg	k Pa
Birth	*	8 - 24	1.1 - 3.2
5 - 10 min	*	33 - 75	4.4 - 10.0
30 min	*	31 - 85	4.1 - 11.3
> 1h	*	55 - 80	7.3 - 10.6
1d	*	54 - 95	7. 2 - 12.6
> 1d	*	83 - 108	11.0 - 14.4

Specimen Type:	Arterial Whole Blood
Reference:	Behrman RE, Ed. Nelson textbook of pediatrics, 14th ed. Philadelphia, PA: WB Saunders Company, 1992, p 1818.
Method(s):	Not given.
Comments:	*Numbers not provided.

OXYGEN SATURATION

		Male and Female	
Age	n	%	Saturated Fraction
Newborn	*	85 - 90	0.85 - 0.90
Thereafter	*	95 - 99	0.95 - 0.99

Specimen Type:	Arterial Whole Blood
Reference:	Behrman RE, Ed. Nelson textbook of pediatrics, 14th ed. Philadelphia, PA: WB Saunders Company, 1992, p 1818.
Method(s):	Not given.
Comments:	*Numbers not provided.

PARATHYROID HORMONE
(PTH)

Age	n	Male and Female pg/mL
Mid-Molecule (C-Terminal)		
1 - 16y	39	51 - 217
Adults	100	50 - 330
N-Terminal Specific		
2 - 13y	18	14 - 21
Adults	200	8 - 24
Intact (IRMA)		
Cord blood	20	≤ 3.0
2 - 20y	150	9 - 52
Adults	200	10 - 65

Specimen Type:	Serum
Reference:	Nichols Institute. Pediatric Endocrine Testing, 1993:31-2.
Method(s):	IRMA - Immunoradiometric assay N-terminal Specific - Radioimmunoassay C-Terminal - Radioimmunoassay
Comments:	Results are 2.5 - 97.5th percentiles.

pH

Test	Age	n	Male and Female
1.	0 – 1mo	200	7.18 - 7.51
	1 – 6mo	100	7.18 - 7.50
	6 – 12mo	85	7.27 - 7.49
2.	Cord Blood[a]	169	7.26 - 7.50
	2 – 5d[b]	28	7.30 - 7.49

Specimen Type:	1,2 Whole blood
Reference:	1. Snell J, Greeley C, Colaco A, et al. Pediatric reference ranges for arterial pH, whole blood electrolytes and glucose. Clin Chem 1993;39:1173. (Abstract) 2. a. Dickman KA. In: Meites S, Ed. Pediatric clinical chemistry, 3rd ed. Washington, DC: AACC Press, 1989:24-5. b. Lockitch G, Halstead AC. In: Meites S, Ed. Pediatric clinical chemistry, 3rd ed. Washington, DC: AACC Press, 1989:25.
Method:	1. Ion specific electrode. (Ciba Corning 288 blood gas system. Ciba Corning Diagnostics, East Walpole, MA.) 2. a. Ion specific electrode. (IL-813, Instrumentation Laboratories, Lexington, MA.) b. Ion specific electrode. (Nova Biomedical Stat Profile, Nova Biomedical, Waltham, MA.)
Comments:	1. Study used hospitalized patients and a computerized approach to removing outliers. Values are 2.5 - 97.5th percentiles. 2. a. In-house study of newborns with Apgar scores of 7 or more. b. Healthy term infants. Mean birth weight 3465g. Results are 2.5 - 97.5th percentiles.

PHOSPHORUS

Test	Age	n	mg/dL	mmol/L	n	mg/dL	mmol/L
			Male			**Female**	
1.	1 - 30d	62	3.9 - 6.9	1.25 - 2.25	66	4.3 - 7.7	1.40 - 2.50
	31 - 365d	83	3.5 - 6.6	1.15 - 2.15	66	3.7 - 6.5	1.20 - 2.10
	1 - 3y	126	3.1 - 6.0	1.00 - 1.95	119	3.4 - 6.0	1.10 - 1.95
	4 - 6y	112	3.3 - 5.6	1.05 - 1.80	107	3.2 - 5.5	1.05 - 1.80
	7 - 9y	117	3.0 - 5.4	0.95 - 1.75	107	3.1 - 5.5	1.00 - 1.80
	10 - 12y	135	3.2 - 5.7	1.05 - 1.85	115	3.3 - 5.3	1.05 - 1.70
	13 - 15y	109	2.9 - 5.1	0.95 - 1.65	110	2.8 - 4.8	0.90 - 1.55
	16 - 18y	95	2.7 - 4.9	0.85 - 1.60	122	2.5 - 4.8	0.80 - 1.55
2.	0 - 5d (< 2.5 kg)	50	4.6 - 8.0	1.50 - 2.60	50	4.6 - 8.0	1.50 - 2.60
	1 - 3y	50	3.9 - 6.5	1.25 - 2.10	50	3.9 - 6.5	1.25 - 2.10
	4 - 6y	38	4.0 - 5.4	1.30 - 1.75	38	4.0 - 5.4	1.30 - 1.75
	7 - 9y	72	3.7 - 5.6	1.20 - 1.80	72	3.7 - 5.6	1.20 - 1.80
	10 - 11y	62	3.7 - 5.6	1.20 - 1.80	62	3.7 - 5.6	1.20 - 1.80
	12 - 13y	73	3.3 - 5.4	1.05 - 1.75	73	3.3 - 5.4	1.05 - 1.75
	14 - 15y	91	2.9 - 5.4	0.95 - 1.75	91	2.9 - 5.4	0.95 - 1.75
	16 - 19y	107	2.8 - 4.6	0.90 - 1.50	107	2.8 - 4.6	0.90 - 1.50
3.	0 - 30d	181	2.7 – 7.2	0.87 - 2.33	140	3.0 - 8.0	0.97 - 2.58
	31 – 90d	84	3.0 – 6.8	0.97 – 2.20	87	3.0 – 7.5	0.97 – 2.42
	3 – 12mo	109	3.0 – 6.9	0.97 – 2.23	119	2.5 – 7.0	0.81 – 2.26
	13 – 24mo	69	2.5 – 6.4	0.81 – 2.07	78	3.0 – 6.5	0.97 – 2.10
	2 - <13y	148	3.0 – 6.0	0.97 – 1.94	254	2.5 – 6.0	0.81 – 1.94
	13 - <16y	175	3.0 – 5.4	0.97 – 1.74	72	3.0 – 5.6	0.97 – 1.81
	16 - <18y	72	3.0 – 5.2	0.97 – 1.68	196	3.0 – 4.8	0.97 - 1.55

Specimen:	1,2,3. Serum or Plasma
Reference:	1. Soldin SJ, Hicks JM, Bailey J, et al. Pediatric reference ranges for phosphate on the Hitachi 747 analyzer. Clin Chem 1997;43:S198. (Abstract)
	2. Lockitch G, Halstead AC, Albersheim S, et al. Age and sex specific pediatric reference intervals for biochemistry analytes as measured with the Ektachem 700 analyzer. Clin Chem 1988;34:1622-5.
	3. Soldin SJ, Hunt C, Hicks JM. Pediatric reference ranges for Phosphorus on the Vitros 500 Analyzer. Clin Chem 1999;45:A22. (Abstract)
Method:	1. Hitachi 747 using ammonium molybdate method (Boehringer-Mannheim, Diagnostics, Indianapolis, IN).
	2,3. Ektachem 700 (2) and 500 (3) using ammonium molybdate method. (Johnson & Johnson, Rochester, NY.)
Comments:	1,3. Study used hospitalized patients and a computerized approach to removing outliers. Values are 2.5 - 97.5th percentiles.
	2. Study used normal healthy children. Values are 2.5 - 97.5th percentiles.

POTASSIUM

Test	Age	n	Male and Female mmol/L
1.	0 - 1wk	100	3.2 - 5.5
	1wk - 1mo	100	3.4 - 6.0
	1 - 6mo	100	3.5 - 5.6
	6mo - 1y	100	3.5 - 6.1
	over 1y	105	3.3 - 4.6
2.	1 - 15y	*	3.7 - 5.0
	16y - Adult	*	3.7 - 4.8
3.	0 - 1mo	207	2.5 - 5.4
	1 - 6mo	96	2.7 - 5.2

Specimen Type:	1, 2 Plasma 3. Whole Blood
Reference:	1. Greeley C, Snell J, Colaco A, et al. Pediatric reference ranges for electrolytes and creatinine. Clin Chem 1993;39:1172. (Abstract) 2. Burritt MF, Slockbower JM, Forsman BS, et al. Pediatric reference intervals for 19 biologic variables in healthy children. Mayo Clinic Proceedings 1990;65:329-36. 3. Snell J, Greeley C, Colaco A, et al. Pediatric reference ranges for arterial pH, whole blood electrolytes, and glucose. Clin Chem 1993;39:1173. (Abstract)
Method(s):	1. Ektachem 700 (Johnson & Johnson, Rochester, NY). 2. Flame Photometry - American Monitor (American Diagnostics, Inc., Indianapolis, IN). 3. 288 Blood Gas System (Ciba Corning Diagnostics, East Walpole, MA).
Comments:	1. Study used hospitalized patients and a computerized approach to removing outliers. 2. From normal healthy children. *See reference for numbers. 3. Study used hospitalized patients and a computerized approach to removing outliers. All of the above values are 2.5 - 97.5th percentiles.

PREALBUMIN
(TRANSTHYRETIN)

Test	Age		Male and Female		
		n	mg/L	mg/dL	
1.	0 - 1mo	63	70 - 390	7.0 - 39.0	
	1 - 6mo	55	83 - 340	8.3 - 34.0	
	6mo - 4y	159	20 - 360	2.0 - 36.0	
	4 - 6y	59	120 - 300	12.0 - 30.0	
	6 - 19y	189	120 - 420	12.0 - 42.0	
2.	0 - 5d	69	60 - 210	6.0 - 21.0	
	1 - 5y	68	140 - 300	14.0 - 30.0	
	6 - 9y	68	150 - 330	15.0 - 33.0	
	10 - 13y	61	200 - 360	20.0 - 36.0	
	14 - 19y	70	220 - 450	22.0 - 45.0	
3.	0 - 4d	118	73 - 144	7.3 - 14.4	
	1mo - 4y	116	67 - 171	6.7 - 17.1	
	5 - 11y	149	91 - 220	9.1 - 22.0	
	12 - 20y	207	124 - 302	12.4 - 30.2	

Specimen Type:	1,2,3 Serum
Reference:	1. Davis ML, Austin C, Messmer BL, et al. IFCC-standardized pediatric reference intervals for 10 serum proteins using the Beckman Array 360 system. Clin Biochem 1996;29:489-92.
	2. Lockitch G, Halstead AZ, Quigley G, et al. Age and sex specific pediatric reference intervals: study design and methods illustrated by measurement of serum proteins with the Behring LN Nephelometer. Clin Chem 1988;34:1618-21.
	3. Hamlin CR, Pankowsky DA. Turbidimetric determination of transthyretin (Prealbumin) with a centrifugal analyzer. Clin Chem 1987;33:144-6.
Method(s):	1. Rate nephelometry. Beckman Array 360 (Beckman Instruments, Brea, CA.).
	2. Nephelometry using the Behring LN Nephelometer (Behring Diagnostics, Westwood MA).
	3. Immunoturbidimetric procedure using a Cobas-Bio centrifugal analyzer (Roche Analytical Instruments, Inc., Nutley, NJ) and rabbit antiserum (Behring Diagnostics, La Jolla, CA).
Comments:	1. Samples were obtained from children attending outpatient clinics. Results are 2.5 - 97.5th percentiles.
	2. No significant differences were found for males and females. These ranges were therefore derived from combined data. The study used healthy children. Results are 2.5 - 97.5th percentiles.
	3. Healthy children. Values are 2.5 - 97.5th percentiles.

PROGESTERONE

Age	Male			Female		
	n	ng/dL	nmol/L	n	ng/dL	nmol/L
6 - 9y	23*	≤ 20	≤ 64	23*	≤ 20	<0.64
10 - 11y	25*	≤ 20	≤ 64	25*	≤ 20	<0. 64
12 - 17y	24	≤ 20 for males	≤ 64			
Adult males	**	10 - 50	32 - 159			
Adult females						
Follicular phase				**	≤ 50	≤ 1.59
Luteal phase				**	300 - 2500	9.54 – 79.50
Postmenopausal				**	≤ 40	≤ 1.27
Pregnancy 1st trimester				**	725 - 4400	23.06 – 139.9
2nd trimester				**	1950 - 8250	62.01 – 262.35
3rd trimester				**	6500 - 22,900	206.7 – 728.2

Specimen Type:	Serum
Reference:	Nichols Institute. Pediatric Endocrine Testing, 1993:34.
Method(s):	Extraction, Radioimmunoassay.
Comments:	Results are 2.5 - 97.5th percentiles. *Males and females combined **Numbers not provided.

PROLACTIN

Test	Age	Male		Female	
		n	ng/mL - µg/L	n	ng/mL - µg/L
1.	0 - 1mo	45	3.7 - 81.2	43	0.3 - 95.0
	1 - 12mo	99	0.3 - 28.9	89	0.2 - 29.9
	1 - 3mo	141	2.3 - 13.2	114	1.0 - 17.1
	4 - 6y	106	0.8 - 16.9	139	1.6 - 13.1
	7 - 9y	105	1.9 - 11.6	98	0.3 - 12.9
	10 - 12y	109	0.9 - 12.9	108	1.9 - 9.6
	13 - 15y	138	1.6 - 16.6	122	3.0 - 14.4
	16 - 18y	95	2.7 - 15.2	104	2.1 - 18.4
2.	< 2y	158	2.7 - 25.0	41	4.2 - 20.2
	2 - 5y	142	1.7 - 17.0	91	1.0 - 17.5
	6 - 10y	103	0.7 - 15.8	140	1.2 - 15.5
	11 - 20y	91	2.0 - 18.2	280	1.5 - 19.5
3.	< 2y	158	2.3 - 18.3	41	3.3 - 14.7
	2 - 5y	142	1.6 - 12.5	91	1.0 - 12.8
	6 - 10y	103	0.8 - 11.6	140	1.2 - 11.4
	11 - 20y	91	1.8 - 13.3	280	1.4 - 14.3

Specimen Type: 1,2,3 Plasma, Serum

Reference:

1. Cook JF, Hicks JM, Godwin ID, et al. Pediatric reference ranges for prolactin. (Abstract.) Clin Chem 1992;38:959.

2. Soldin SJ, Morales A, Albalos F, et al. Pediatric reference ranges the Abbott IMx analyzer for FSH, LH, prolactin TSH, T_4, T_3, free T_4, free T_3, T-uptake, IgE and ferritin. Clin Biochem 1995;28:603-6.

3. Murthy JN, Hicks JM, Soldin SJ. Evaluation of the Technicon Immuno I Random Access Immunoassay Analyzer and calculation of pediatric reference ranges for endocrine tests, T-uptake, and ferritin. Clin Biochem 1995;28:181-5.

Method(s):

1. Hybritech Tandem Prolactin procedure. (Hybritech Inc, San Diego, CA.)

2. IMx Analyzer (Abbott Laboratories, Abbott Park, IL).

3. Immuno I (Bayer Corp., Tarrytown, NY).

Comments: 1,2,3 Studies used hospitalized patients and a computerized approach adapted from the Hoffmann technique. Values are 2.5 - 97.5th percentiles.

PROTEIN, TOTAL

Test	Age	Male			Female		
		n	g/dL	g/L	n	g/dL	g/L
1.	1 – 60d	62	3.9 – 7.6	39 – 76	69	3.4 – 7.0	34 – 70
	61 – 180d	130	4.1 – 7.9	41 - 79	161	3.9 – 7.6	39 - 76
	181d – 1y	268	3.9 – 7.9	39 - 79	196	4.5 – 7.8	45 - 78
2.	0 - 5d (< 2.5 kg)	30	3.8 - 6.2	38 - 62	30	3.8 - 6.2	38 - 62
	0 - 5d (> 2.5 kg)	93	5.4 - 7.0	54 - 70	93	5.4 - 7.0	54 - 70
	1 - 3y	50	5.9 - 7.0	59 - 70	50	5.9 - 7.0	59 - 70
	4 - 6y	38	5.9 - 7.8	59 - 78	38	5.9 - 7.8	59 - 78
	7 - 9y	74	6.2 - 8.1	62 - 81	74	6.2 - 8.1	62 - 81
	10 – 19y	332	6.3 - 8.6	63 - 86	332	6.3 - 8.6	63 - 86
3.	1 – 30d	68	4.1 - 6.3	41 - 63	51	4.2 - 6.2	42 - 62
	31 – 182d	58	4.7 - 6.7	47 - 67	42	4.4 - 6.6	44 - 66
	183 – 365d	29	5.5 - 7.0	55 - 70	186	5.6 - 7.9	56 - 79
	1 – 18y	652	5.7 - 8.0	57 - 80	440	5.7 - 8.0	57 - 80

Specimen Type:	1, 3. Serum/Plasma
	2. Plasma
Reference:	1. Soldin SJ, Morse AS. Pediatric Reference Ranges for Albumin and Total Protein in Children <1 Year Old Using the Vitros 500 Analyzer. Clin Chem 1998; 44:A15. (Abstract)
	2. Lockitch G, Halstead AC, Albersheim S, et al. Age and sex specific pediatric reference intervals for biochemistry analytes as measured with the Ektachem 700 analyzer. Clin Chem 1988;34:1622-5.
	3. Hicks JM, Bjorn S, Beatey J, et al. Pediatric reference ranges for albumin, globulin and total protein on the Hitachi 747. Clin Chem 1995;41:S93. (Abstract)
Method(s):	1. Vitros 500
	2. Biuret method. Ektachem 700 (Johnson & Johnson, Rochester, NY).
	3. Boehringer-Mannheim total protein reagent (Biuret). Total protein was measured on the Hitachi 747. (Boehringer-Mannheim Diagnostics, Indianapolis, IN.)
Comments:	1,3. Study used hospitalized patients and a computerized approach to removing outliers. Values are 2.5 - 97.5th percentiles.
	2. Healthy term and pre-term neonates and normal healthy children. Values are 2.5 - 97.5th percentiles.

PROTEIN CEREBROSPINAL FLUID
(CSF PROTEIN)

Age			Male and Female	
Age	n	mg/dL	mg/L	
Full-term newborn	*	40 - 120	400 - 1200	
< 1 mo	*	20 - 80	200 - 800	
> 1 mo	*	15 - 45	150 - 450	

Specimen Type:	Cerebrospinal fluid
Reference:	Meites S, Ed. Pediatric clinical chemistry, 2nd ed. Washington, DC: AACC Press, 1981:376.
Method(s):	Nephelometry
Comments:	*Numbers not provided.

153

Test	Age	n	mg/dL	µmol/L
			Male and Female	
1.	All ages	*	0.70 - 1.32	80 - 150
2.	All ages	*	0.3 - 0.70	35 - 80

PYRUVATE

Specimen Type:	1,2	Whole blood, proteins precipitated with perchloric acid.
Reference:	1.	Reference values and SI unit information. The Hospital for Sick Children, Toronto, 1993:378.
	2.	Children's National Medical Center, Washington, DC. Unpublished data.
Method(s):	1,2	Standard enzymatic approach.
Comments:	1,2	*Numbers not available.

RENIN (PLASMA)

Age	n	ng/L
1 - 6y	63	6.3 – 149
7 - 12y	68	5.5 – 110
13 - 17y	87	3.3 - 61

Specimen Type:	Plasma
Reference:	Coates JE, Chapelski LJ, Yatscoff RW. Pediatric reference intervals for plasma renin. Clin Biochem 1994;27:316-7.
Method(s):	Renin Active Pasteur CT kits (Sanofi Diagnostics Pasteur, Inc., Montreal, Quebec, Canada)
Comments:	Children seen as outpatients were tested. Male and female ranges were not significantly different and they were combined for calculations of the above ranges. The results reported are 2.5 - 97.5th percentiles.

RENIN ACTIVITY

Age	n	Male and Female ng/mL/h
0 - 1w	7	0 - 40
2 - 4w	7	0 - 175
3mo - 1y	*	≤ 15
1 - 4y	*	≤ 10
4 - 15y	*	≤ 6

Specimen Type:	Plasma
Reference:	Nichols Institute. Pediatric Endocrine Testing, 1993:33.
Method(s):	Radioimmunoassay.
Comments:	Normal sodium diet. Patients over 1y of age were supine from 9 - 11 am before specimens were drawn.
	*Numbers not provided.

RETINOL BINDING PROTEIN
(RBP)

Test	Age	n	Male and Female mg/dL	Male and Female µmol/L
1.	0 - 5d	64	0.8 - 4.5	0.38 - 2.15
	1 - 5y	68	1.0 - 7.6	0.48 - 3.62
	6 - 9y	64	2.0 - 7.8	0.95 - 3.72
	10 - 13y	59	1.3 - 9.9	0.62 - 4.72
	14 - 19y	70	3.0 - 9.2	1.43 - 4.39
2.	Mothers	25	3.6 - 10.7	1.72 - 5.12
	Infants	25	1.7 - 7.3	0.83 - 3.47
3.	Term Neonates (> 37 wk)	41	1.02 - 3.14	0.49 - 1.51
	Preterm Neonates (< 36.6 wk)	58	0.72 - 2.88	0.35 - 1.38

Specimen Type:
1,2 Serum
3. Serum, Plasma

Reference:

1. Lockitch G, Halstead AZ, Quigley G, et al. Age and sex specific pediatric reference intervals: study design and methods illustrated by measurement of serum proteins with the Behring LN Nephelometer. Clin Chem 1988;34:1618-21.

2. Jansson L, Nilsson B. Serum retinol and retinol binding protein in mothers and infants at delivery. Biol Neonate 1983;43:269-71.

3. Cardona-Pérez A, et al. Cord blood retinol and retinol binding protein in preterm and term neonates. Nutrition Research 1996:16;191-6.

Method(s):

1. Nephelometry using the Behring LN Nephelometer (Behring Diagnostics, Westwood MA).

2. Electroimmunoassay. A rabbit antiserum against human RBP was used.

3. Radial Immunodiffusion (Behring Diagnostics, La Jolla, CA.)

Comments:

1. No significant differences were found for males and females. These ranges were therefore derived from combined data. The study used healthy children. Results are 2.5 - 97.5th percentiles.

2. The study population consisted of 25 healthy term infants and their mothers. Results are mean ± 2SD.

3. Healthy term and preterm neonates studied. Results are 2.5 - 97.5th percentiles.

REVERSE TRIIODOTHYRONINE (rT₃)			

		Male and Female	
Age	n	ng/dL	nmol/L
1 - 5y	*	15 - 71	0.23 - 1.10
5 - 10y	*	17 - 79	0.26 - 1.20
10 - 15y	*	19 - 88	0.29 - 1.36
Adults	*	30 - 80	0.46 - 1.23

Specimen Type:	Serum.
Reference:	Behrman RE, Ed. Nelson textbook of pediatrics, 14th ed. Philadelphia, PA: WB Saunders Company, 1992, p 1821.
Method(s):	Not given.
Comments:	*Numbers not provided.

SELENIUM

Test	Age	n	Male and Female	
			μg/dL	μmol/L
1.	0 - 5d*	20	6 - 9	0.72 - 1.20
	1 - 5y*	30	10 - 14	1.22 - 1.82
	6 - 9y*	30	10 - 16	1.29 - 2.05
	10 – 14y*	30	10 - 19	1.31 - 2.35
	15 – 19y*	27	10 - 19	1.31 - 2.35
2.	3 – 5y	38	2.0 - 12.4	0.25 - 1.57
	6 – 8y	43	1.6 - 12.0	0.20 - 1.52
	9 – 11y	52	2.4 – 13.5	0.30 - 1.70
	12 – 13y	24	4.0 - 10.7	0.51 - 1.35
	14 – 16y	29	4.0 - 10.7	0.51 - 1.35
3.	0 – <0.5y	13	0.8 – 4.4	0.10 – 0.58
	0.5 – <1.0y	18	0 – 6.9	0.00 – 0.87
	1.0 – <2.0y	15	1.5 – 7.3	0.20 – 0.96
	2.0 – <4.0y	23	0.9 – 10.4	0.12 – 1.36
	4.0 – <6.0y	19	0.6 – 12.5	0.08 – 1.64
	6.0 – <10.0y	25	2.4 – 11.8	0.31 – 1.55
	10.0 – <14.0y	21	2.4 – 11.4	0.30 – 1.50
	14.0 – <18.0y	17	2.1 – 11.8	0.27 – 1.55

| Specimen Type: | 1, 2. | Serum |
| | 3. | Serum/Plasma |

Reference:	1.	Lockitch G, Halstead A, Wadsworth L, et al. Age and sex specific pediatric reference intervals for zinc, copper, selenium, iron, vitamins A and E and related proteins. Clin Chem 1988;34:1625-8.
	2.	Malvy DJ-M, Arnaud J, Burtschy B, et al. Reference values for serum, zinc and selenium of French healthy children. Eur J Epidemiol 1993;9:155-61.
	3.	Rükgauer M, Klein J, Kruse-Jarres JD. Reference Values for the Trace Elements Copper, Manganese, Selenium, and Zinc in the Serum/Plasma of Children, Adolescents, and Adults. J Trace Elements Med Biol 1997;11:92-8

Method(s):	1.	Varian GTA - 95. Atomic absorption. (Varian Canada, Inc., Georgetown, Ontario, Canada.)
	2.	Perkin-Elmer atomic absorption spectrophotometry (Perkin-Elmer Corporation, Norwalk, CT).
	3.	Atomic Absorption Spectrophotometry with Zeeman backgroung compensation. Perkin Elmer ETAAS, Zeeman 3030, Uberlingen, Germany

| Comments: | 1. | The study population was healthy children. Non-parametric methods were used to determine the 0.025 and 0.975 fractiles.

*No significant differences were found for males and females. These ranges were therefore derived from combined data. |
| | 2. | The study population consisted of healthy French children. Values reported are the 2.5 - 97.5th percentiles.

Note: Reference ranges differ greatly on a geographic basis. Data must be interpreted against locally derived reference ranges. |
| | 3. | Study population was drawn from patients visiting the outpatient department or surgical or orthopedic ward for preoperative work up. Results are mean ±2 SDs (2.5th – 97.5th percentiles). |

SERUM OSTEOCALCIN

Age, years	Male		Female	
	n	μg/L	n	μg/L
1	43	52-63	31	48-79
2	24	64-70	31	61-88
3	39	54-70	35	44-93
4	43	53-90	47	51-98
5	55	52-83	49	66-88
6	59	51-84	66	65-96
7	51	49-104	42	53-97
8	66	51-80	78	50-89
9	70	62-83	57	61-78
10	86	58-88	82	65-96
11	78	56-80	69	36-93
12	41	68-80	39	74-99
13	47	74-98	35	42-75
14	55	66-102	51	25-43
15	49	61-105	50	35-59
16	27	36-50	39	27-47

Specimen Type:	Serum
Reference:	Cioffi M, Molinari AM, Gazzero P, et al. Serum osteocalcin in 1634 healthy children. Clin Chem 1997;43:543-5.
Method(s):	Sandwich IRMA (Osteo-ELSA; CIS Bio International, Gif sur Yvette, France)
Comments:	Study used 1634 healthy children. Results are 25th and 75th percentiles. Osteocalcin is an important marker of bone turnover.

161

SEX HORMONE BINDING GLOBULIN
(SHBG)

Test	Age	Male			Female		
		n	nmol/L	µg/dL	n	nmol/L	µg/dL
1.	1 - 30d	57	10.8 - 70.8	0.31 - 2.04	49	11.8 - 51.4	0.34 - 1.48
	31 - 365d	93	60.2 - 208.5	1.73 - 6.01	68	50.4 - 181.2	1.45 - 5.22
	1 - 3y	109	42.4 - 155.6	1.22 - 4.48	98	51.4 - 157.7	1.48 - 4.54
	4 - 6y	75	39.4 - 145.6	1.14 - 4.20	73	47.8 - 142.1	1.38 - 4.10
	7 - 9y	70	37.7 - 114.4	1.09 - 3.30	29	31.0 - 103.0	0.89 - 2.97
	10 - 12y	113	31.6 - 92.5	0.91 - 2.67	60	20.0 - 99.6	0.58 - 2.87
	13 - 15y	78	13.3 - 62.6	0.38 - 1.80	80	16.6 - 76.5	0.48 - 2.20
	16 - 18y	34	10.6 - 53.6	0.31 - 1.54	39	9.3 - 75.2	0.27 - 2.17

Specimen Type:	Serum or Plasma
Reference:	Soldin SJ, Hicks JM, Bailey J, et al. Pediatric reference ranges for sex hormone binding globulin. Clin Chem 1997;43:S200. (Abstract)
Method(s):	Time-resolved fluoroimmunoassay. Delfia SHBG kit (Wallac Oy, Turku, Finland)
Comments:	Study used hospitalized patients and a computerized adaptation of the Hoffmann technique. Values are 2.5 - 97.5th percentiles.

SODIUM

Test	Age	n	Male and Female mmol/L
1.	0 - 7d	100	133 - 146
	7 - 31d	100	134 - 144
	1 - 6mo	100	134 - 142
	6mo - 1y	100	133 - 142
	> 1y	105	134 - 143
2.	0 - 1mo	59	127 - 143
	2 - 6mo	49	130 - 147

Specimen Type:	1.	Plasma
	2.	Heparinized Whole Blood
Reference:	1.	Greeley C, Snell J, Colaco A, et al. Pediatric reference ranges for electrolytes and creatinine. Clin Chem 1993;39:1172. (Abstract)
	2.	Snell J, Greeley C, Colaco A, et al. Pediatric reference ranges for arterial pH, whole blood electrolytes and glucose. Clin Chem 1993;39:1173. (Abstract)
Method(s):	1.	Kodak Ektachem 700 analyzer. (Johnson & Johnson, Rochester, NY).
	2.	Corning 288 Blood Gas System. (Ciba-Corning Diagnostics, East Walpole, MA).
Comments:	1.	Study used hospitalized patients and a computerized approach adapted from the Hoffmann technique to obtain the 2.5 - 97.5th percentiles.
	2.	Study used hospitalized patients and a computerized approach adapted from the Hoffmann technique to obtain the 2.5 - 97.5th percentiles.

SWEAT ELECTROLYTES

Test	Age	n	Male and Female mmol/L	mmol/L
			chloride	sodium
1.	1wk – Adult	*	< 40	< 40
	Patients with cystic fibrosis	*	> 60	> 60
2.	0 - 3.9mo	170	6 - 40	4 - 40
	4 - 11.9mo	70	4 - 29	5 - 39
	1 - 4.9y	134	6 - 54	6 - 54
	5 - 11.9y	45	8 - 65	8 - 65
	> 12y	23	11 - 77	11 - 77

Specimen Type:	1,2	Sweat
Reference:	1.	Children's National Medical Center. Unpublished data.
	2.	Meites S, Ed. Pediatric clinical chemistry, 3rd ed. Washington, DC: AACC Press, 1989:246.
Method(s):	1.	Pilocarpine iontophoresis/macroduct collection. Measured on Ektachem 500 (Johnson & Johnson, Rochester, NY). Cl measured on Chloridometer (Radiometer, Cleveland, OH).
	2.	Pilocarpine iontophoresis. Flame photometry for sodium, chloridometer for chloride.
Comments:	1.	Results between 40-60 mmol/L require repeat testing and or use of other tests such as immunoreactive trypsin, bentiromide test of pancreatic function, and DNA probe test for CF gene.
		*Numbers not provided.
	2.	Based on in-house studies of non-affected individuals.

TESTOSTERONE

Age	Male			Female		
	n	ng/dL	nmol/L	n	ng/dL	nmol/L
1 - 5mo	10	1 - 177	0.03 - 6.14	5	1 - 5	0.03 - 0.17
6 - 11mo	8	2 - 7	0.07 - 0.24	6	2 - 5	0.07 - 0.17
1 - 5y	16	2 - 25	0.07 - 0.87	17	2 - 10	0.07 - 0.35
6 - 9y	30	3 - 30	0.10 - 1.04	16	2 - 20	0.07 - 0.35
10 - 11y	20	5 - 50	0.17 - 1.73	10	5 - 25	0.17 - 0.87
12 - 14y	28	10 - 572	0.35 - 19.83	17	10 - 40	0.35 - 1.39
15 - 17y	18	220 - 800	7.63 - 27.74	11	5 - 40	0.17 - 1.39
Adults	*	280 - 1100	9.71 - 38.14	*	15 - 70	0.52 - 2.43

Specimen Type:	Serum
Reference:	Nichols Institute. Pediatric Endocrine Testing, 1993:38.
Method(s):	Extraction, Chromatography, Radioimmunoassay.
Comments:	Results are 2.5 - 97.5th percentiles. *Numbers not provided.

THYROID STIMULATING HORMONE
(TSH)

Test	Age	n	Male µU/mL mU/L	n	Female µU/mL mU/L
1.	0 - 1mo	84	< 6.5	62	< 6.0
	1 - 12mo	114	< 4.1	103	< 4.0
	1 - 3y	128	< 3.0	126	< 3.3
	4 - 6y	109	< 3.0	82	< 2.8
	7 - 12y	112	< 3.1	107	< 2.9
	13 - 18y	106	< 3.1	106	< 3.0
2.	1 - 30d	63	0.52 - 16.00	89	0.72 - 13.10
	1mo - 5y	95	0.55 - 7.10	95	0.46 - 8.10
	6 - 18y	95	0.37 - 6.00	96	0.36 - 5.80
3.	1 - 30d	63	0.76 - 16.11	89	0.96 - 13.68
	1mo - 5y	95	0.80 - 7.52	95	0.70 - 8.55
	6 - 18y	95	0.61 - 6.39	96	0.60 - 6.18
4.			Male and Female		
	Age	n	mU/L (µU/mL)		
	0 - <2y	36	0.668 – 4.465		
	2 - <7y	149	0.400 – 3.200		
	7 - <13y	128	0.300 – 2.689		
	13 - <18y	123	0.400 – 1.900		

Specimen Type:	1,2,3,4. Plasma, Serum
Reference:	1. Hicks JM, Godwin ID, Beatey J, et al. Pediatric reference ranges for highly sensitive TSH. Clin Chem 1992;38:960. (Abstract)
	2. Soldin SJ, Morales A, Albalos F, et al. Pediatric reference ranges on the Abbott IMx for FSH, LH, prolactin, TSH, T_4, T_3, free T_4, free T_3, T-uptake, IgE and ferritin. Clin Biochem 1995;28:603-6.
	3. Murthy JN, Hicks JM, Soldin SJ. Evaluation of the Technicon Immuno I Random Access Immunoassay Analyzer and calculation of pediatric reference ranges for endocrine tests, T-uptake, and ferritin. Clin Biochem 1995;28:181-5.
	4. Soldin SJ, Hicks JM, Bailey J, et al. Pediatric Reference Ranges for 3rd Generation TSH on the ACS 180. Clin Chem 1998; 44:A13 (Abstract).
Method(s):	1. Delphia Immunofluorescent TSH Kit (Pharmacia ENI Diagnostics Inc., Columbia, MD).
	2. Abbott IMx analyzer (Abbott Laboratories, Abbott Park, IL).
	3. Immuno I (Bayer Corp., Tarrytown, NY).
	4. ACS 180 using Chiron Diagnostics TSH-3kit. (Chiron Diagnostics Corp., East Walpole, MA)
Comments:	1. Study used hospitalized patients and a computerized approach adapted from the Hoffmann technique. Values are 97.5th percentile. Lower limit of detection 0.1 µU/mL.
	2,3 Study used hospitalized patients and a computerized approach adapted from the Hoffmann technique. Values are 2.5 - 97.5th percentiles. Lower limit of detection 0.03 µU/mL.
	4. Study used hospitalized patients and a computerized approach adapted from the Hoffmann technic. Values are 2.5 – 97.5th percentiles. Lower limit of detection 0.003 µU/mL.

THYROXINE BINDING GLOBULIN
(TBG)

Test	Age	Male n	Male mg/L	Female n	Female mg/L
1.	1 - 12mo	189	16.2 - 32.9	138	17.7 - 32.0
	1 - 3y	167	16.4 - 32.0	112	19.3 - 33.8
	4 - 6y	100	16.6 - 29.8	91	18.3 - 30.8
	7 - 12y	184	16.5 - 28.8	133	15.0 - 29.2
	13 - 18y	158	13.4 - 25.6	130	13.7 - 28.7
2.	Cord Blood	*	19 - 39	*	19 - 39
	1 - 11mo	*	16 - 36	*	17 - 37
	1 - 9y	*	12 - 28	*	15 - 27
	10 - 19y	*	14 - 26	*	14 - 30

Specimen Type:	1. Plasma 2. Serum or Plasma
Reference:	1. Hicks JM, Godwin ID, Beatey J, et al. Pediatric reference ranges for thyroid binding globulin. Clin Chem 1993:39;1172. (Abstract) 2. Levy RP, Marshall JS, Velayo NL. Radioimmunoassay of human thyroxine binding globulin (TBG). J Clin Endocrinol Metab 1971:32; 372-81.
Method(s):	1. Corning TBG[125] I-Radioimmunoassay. (Ciba Corning Diagnostics Corp., Medfield, MA). 2. Direct RIA using goat antihuman TBG and ^{125}I-labeled human TBG. A second antibody is used for the bound/free separation phase.
Comments:	1. Study used hospitalized patients and a computerized approach to removing outliers. Values are 2.5 - 97.5th percentiles. 2. Study used healthy children. *For numbers at each age group, see Meites S, Ed. Pediatric clinical chemistry, 3rd ed. Washington, DC: AACC Press, 1989:254.

THYROXINE (T₄)

Test	Age	Male n	Male µg/dL	Male nmol/L	Female n	Female µg/dL	Female nmol/L
1.	1 - 30d	108	3.0 - 14.4	39 - 185	116	3.0 - 13.4	39 - 172
	1 - 12mo	98	5.3 - 16.3	68 - 210	95	4.6 - 13.4	59 - 172
	1 - 5y	151	5.5 - 11.4	71 - 147	197	6.3 - 12.8	81 - 165
	6 - 10y	151	5.4 - 10.6	69 - 136	146	5.3 - 10.8	68 - 139
	11 - 15y	171	4.5 - 10.3	58 - 133	160	4.9 - 10.0	63 - 129
	16 - 18y	141	4.9 - 8.8	63 - 113	143	5.1 - 10.0	66 - 129
2.	1 - 30d	100	5.9 - 21.5	76 - 276	106	6.3 - 21.5	81 - 276
	31 - 364d	107	6.4 - 13.9	82 - 179	96	4.9 - 13.7	63 - 176
	1 - 3y	149	7.0 - 13.1	90 - 169	132	7.1 - 14.1	91 - 180
	4 - 6y	139	6.1 - 12.6	79 - 162	117	7.2 - 14.0	93 - 180
	7 - 12y	129	6.7 - 13.4	86 - 172	134	6.1 - 12.1	79 - 156
	13 - 15y	145	4.8 - 11.5	62 - 148	108	5.8 - 11.2	75 - 144
	16 - 18y	49	5.9 - 11.5	76 - 148	112	5.2 - 13.2	67 - 170
3.	1 - 30d	108	3.4 - 12.6	44 - 163	116	3.4 - 11.8	44 - 152
	1 - 12mo	98	5.4 - 14.1	68 - 182	95	4.7 - 11.8	60 - 152
	1 - 5y	151	5.3 - 10.2	69 - 131	197	6.0 - 11.3	78 - 146
	6 - 10y	151	5.3 - 9.5	69 - 122	146	5.2 - 9.7	67 - 125
	11 - 15y	171	4.6 - 9.2	59 - 119	160	4.9 - 9.0	63 - 116
	16 - 18y	141	4.9 - 8.1	63 - 104	143	5.1 - 9.0	66 - 116

Specimen Type: 1,2,3 Plasma, Serum

Reference:

1. Soldin SJ, Morales A, Albalos F, et al. Pediatric reference ranges on the Abbott IMx analyzer for FSH, LH, prolactin, TSH, T₄, T₃, free T₄, free T₃, T-uptake, IgE and ferritin. Clin Biochem 1995;28:603-6.

2. Soldin SJ, Cook J, Beatey J, et al. Pediatric reference ranges for thyroxine and triiodothyronine uptake. Clin Chem 1992;38:960. (Abstract)

3. Murthy JN, Hicks JM, Soldin SJ. Evaluation of the Technicon Immuno I Random Access Immunoassay Analyzer and calculation of pediatric reference ranges for endocrine tests, T-uptake, and ferritin. Clin Biochem 1995;28:181-5.

Method(s):

1. Abbott IMx Analyzer. (Abbott Diagnostics, Inc., Abbott Park, IL.)

2. T₄: Gamma Coat TM[125] (Baxter-Travenol Diagnostics, Inc., Cambridge, MA.)

3. Immuno I (Bayer Corp., Tarrytown, NY)

Comments: 1,2,3 Study used hospitalized patients and a computerized approach adapted from the Hoffmann technique. Values are 2.5 - 97.5th percentiles.

THYROXINE, FREE (FREE T₄)

Test	Age	Male			Female		
		n	ng/dL	pmol/L	n	ng/dL	pmol/L
1.	1 - 3d	24	0.80 - 2.78	10 - 36	38	0.88 - 1.93	11 - 25
	4 - 30d	73	0.48 - 2.32	6 - 30	62	0.61 - 1.93	8 - 25
	1 - 12mo	52	0.76 - 2.00	10 - 26	54	0.88 - 1.84	11 - 24
	1 - 5y	100	0.90 - 1.59	12 - 21	117	1.02 - 1.72	13 - 22
	6 - 10y	104	0.81 - 1.68	10 - 22	101	0.82 - 1.58	11 - 20
	11 - 15y	101	0.92 - 1.57	12 - 20	100	0.79 - 1.49	10 - 19
	16 - 18y	110	0.92 - 1.53	12 - 20	101	0.83 - 1.44	11 - 19
2.	1 - 3d	24	1.16 - 2.95	15 - 38	38	1.09 - 2.09	14 - 27
	4 - 30d	73	0.78 - 2.25	10 - 29	62	0.85 - 2.09	11 - 27
	1 - 12mo	52	1.00 - 2.17	13 - 28	54	1.09 - 2.02	14 - 26
	1 - 5y	100	1.16 - 1.71	15 - 22	117	1.24 - 1.86	16 - 24
	6 - 10y	104	1.09 - 1.86	14 - 24	101	1.09 - 1.71	14 - 22
	11 - 15y	101	1.16 - 1.71	15 - 22	100	1.00 - 1.63	13 - 21
	16 - 18y	110	1.16 - 1.71	15 - 22	101	1.09 - 1.63	14 - 21

Specimen Type:	1,2 Plasma, Serum
Reference:	1. Soldin SJ,. Morales A, Albalos F, et al. Pediatric reference ranges on the Abbott IMx for FSH, LH, prolactin, TSH, T₄, T₃, free T₄, free T₃, T-uptake, IgE and ferritin. Clin Biochem 1995;28:603-6.
	2. Murthy JN, Hicks, JM, Soldin SJ. Evaluation of the Technicon Immuno I Random Access Immunoassay Analyzer and calculation of pediatric reference ranges for endocrine tests, T-uptake, and ferritin. Clin Biochem 1995;28:181-5.
Method(s):	1. Abbott IMx Analyzer. (Abbott Diagnostics, Inc., Abbott Park, IL.)
	2. Immuno I (Bayer Corp., Tarrytown, NY)
Comments:	1,2 Study used hospitalized patients and a computerized approach adapted from the Hoffmann technique. Values are 2.5 - 97.5th percentiles.

TRANSFERRIN

Test	Age	Male and Female	
		n	g/L
1.	0 - 5d	73	1.43 - 4.46
	1 - 3y	51	2.18 - 3.47
	4 - 6y	39	2.08 - 3.78
	7 - 9y	39	2.25 - 3.61
	10 - 13y	110	2.24 - 4.42
	14 - 19y	78	2.33 - 4.44

Test	Age	Male		Female	
		n	g/L	n	g/L
2.	1 - 30d	41	0.97 - 2.05	36	0.92 - 2.08
	31 – 182d	88	1.06 - 3.25	70	1.28 - 3.09
	183 – 365d	40	1.78 - 3.57	29	1.46 - 3.64
	1 - 3y	157	1.96 - 3.65	142	1.49 - 3.82
	4 - 6y	108	2.02 - 3.50	94	1.74 - 3.99
	7 - 9y	91	1.49 - 3.53	91	1.86 - 3.68
	10 - 12y	85	1.73 - 3.80	105	1.85 - 3.77
	13 - 15y	82	1.71 - 3.74	84	1.93 - 3.91
	16 - 18y	60	1.94 - 3.48	82	1.81 - 4.16

Specimen Type:	1,2	Serum, Plasma
Reference:	1.	Lockitch G, Halstead AC, Quigley G, et al. Age and sex specific pediatric reference intervals: study, design and methods illustrated by measurement of serum proteins with the Behring LN Nephelometer. Clin Chem 1988;34:1618-21.
	2.	Soldin SJ, Hicks JM, Bailey J, et al. Pediatric reference ranges for total iron binding capacity and transferrin. Clin Chem 1997;43:S200. (Abstract)
Method(s):	1.	Nephelometric, Behring LN Nephelometer (Behring Diagnostics, Hoechst, Inc., Montreal, Canada).
	2.	Nephelometric, Behring LN Nephelometer (Behring Diagnostics, Inc., Westwood, MA).
Comments:	1.	Normal healthy children. Values provided are 2.5 - 97.5th percentiles.
	2.	Study used hospitalized patients and a computerized adaptation of the Hoffmann technique. Results are 2.5 - 97.5th percentiles.

TRANSFERRIN SATURATION

Age	Male			Female	
	n			n	
1 - 5y*	44	0.07 - 0.44		44	0.07 - 0.44
6 - 9y*	50	0.17 - 0.42		50	0.17 - 0.42
10 - 14y	31	0.11 - 0.36		40	0.02 - 0.40
14 - 19y	65	0.06 - 0.33		110	0.06 - 0.33

Specimen Type:	Plasma
Reference:	Lockitch G, Halstead AC, Wadsworth L, et al. Age and sex specific pediatric reference intervals and correlations for zinc, copper, selenium, iron, vitamins A and E and related proteins. Clin Chem 1988;34:1625-8.
Method(s):	Transferrin was measured by nephelometry. Behring LN with Behring kit (Behringwerke, Marburg, Germany).
Comments:	The study population was healthy children. Non-parametric methods were used to determine the 0.025 and 0.975 fractiles. *Males and females were not studied separately. Transferrin satur-ation = iron (µmoL/L) ÷ TIBC.

TRIGLYCERIDES

Test	Age	Male			Female		
		n	mmol/L	mg/dL	n	mmol/L	mg/dL
1.	0 – 7d	149	0.24 – 2.06	21 – 182	142	0.32 - 1.88	28 – 166
	8 – 30d	283	0.34 – 2.08	30 - 184	172	0.34 – 1.86	30 – 165
	31 – 90d	247	0.45 – 1.98	40 – 175	171	0.40 – 3.19	35 – 282
	91 – 180d	132	0.51 – 3.29	45 - 291	126	0.57 – 4.01	50 – 355
	181 – 365d	286	0.51 – 5.66	45 - 501	261	0.41 – 4.87	36 - 431
2.	1 - 3y	49*	0.31 - 1.41	27 - 125	49*	0.31 - 1.41	27 - 125
	4 - 6y	38*	0.36 - 1.31	32 - 116	38*	0.36 - 1.31	32 - 116
	7 - 9y	72*	0.32 - 1.46	28 - 129	72*	0.32 - 1.46	28 - 129
	10 - 11y	28	0.27 - 1.55	24 - 137	34	0.44 - 1.58	39 - 140
	12 - 13y	32	0.27 - 1.64	24 - 145	40	0.42 - 1.47	37 - 130
	14 - 15y	39	0.38 - 1.86	34 - 165	50	0.43 - 1.52	38 - 135
	16 - 19y	41	0.38 - 1.58	34 - 140	68	0.42 - 1.58	37 - 140
3.	Cord blood serum arterial	397**	0.10 - 1.04	9 - 92	397**	0.10 - 1.04	9 - 92
	Cord blood serum venous	397**	0.13 - 0.97	12 - 86	397**	0.13 - 0.97	12 - 86
	Adult	***	0.55 - 1.7	49 - 151	***	0.55 - 1.7	49 - 151

Specimen Type:	1.	Serum
	2,3.	Serum/Plasma
Reference:	1.	Soldin SJ, Morse AS. Pediatric Reference Ranges for Calcium and Triglycerides in Children <1 Year Old using the Vitros 500 Analyzer. Clin Chem 1998;44:A16 (Abstract).
	2.	Lockitch G, Halstead AC, Albersheim S, et al. Age and sex specific pediatric reference intervals for biochemistry analytes as measured with the Ektachem 700 analyzer. Clin Chem 1988;34:1622-5.
	3.	Perkins SL, Livesey JF, Belcher J. Reference intervals for 21 clinical chemistry analytes in arterial and venous umbilical cord blood. Clin Chem 1993;39:1041-4.
Method(s):	1,2.	Glycerol phosphate oxidase on Kodak Ektachem 700 analyzer (Johnson & Johnson, Rochester, NY)
	3.	Hitachi 737 with Boehringer-Mannheim reagents (Boehringer-Mannheim Canada, Montreal Canada).
Comments:	1.	The study used plasma/serum obtained from hospitalized patients and employed Chauvenet's criteria to remove outliers and a computerized approach adapted from the Hoffmann technic to obtain the 2.5 – 97.5th percentiles. Fasting samples were not obtained in these neonates and infants which accounts for the somewhat elevated 97.5th percentiles.
	2.	A healthy population of children 1-19y were studied. Results are 2.5 - 97.5th percentiles. *No significant differences were found for males and females. These ranges were therefore derived from combined data.
	3.	Results are 2.5 - 97.5th percentiles. **No significant differences were found for males and females. These ranges were therefore derived from combined data. ***See reference for numbers.

TRIIODOTHYRONINE (T₃)

Test	Age	n	ng/dL	nmol/L	n	ng/dL	nmol/L
		Male			**Female**		
1.	1 - 30d	50	15 - 210	0.2 - 3.2	47	15 - 200	0.2 - 3.1
	1 - 12mo	111	95 - 275	1.5 - 4.2	100	50 - 264	0.8 - 4.1
	1 - 5y	101	80 - 253	1.2 - 3.9	115	126 - 258	1.9 - 4.0
	6 - 10y	99	96 - 232	1.5 - 3.6	99	104 - 227	1.6 - 3.5
	11 - 15y	97	73 - 199	1.1 - 3.1	100	96 - 211	1.5 - 3.2
	16 - 18y	100	69 - 201	1.1 - 3.1	104	91 - 164	1.4 - 2.5
2.	1 - 30d	227	29 - 179	0.4 - 2.7	173	34 - 173	0.5 - 2.7
	1 - 3y	115	58 - 190	0.9 - 2.9	127	54 - 199	0.8 - 3.1
	4 - 6y	112	59 - 177	0.9 - 2.7	105	58 - 173	0.9 - 2.7
	7 - 12y	114	52 - 192	0.8 - 2.9	110	53 - 171	0.8 - 2.6
	13 - 18y	113	64 - 157	1.0 - 2.4	121	40 - 156	0.6 - 2.4
3.	1 - 30d	50	51 - 184	0.7 - 2.9	47	48 - 177	0.7 - 2.8
	1 - 12mo	111	103 - 229	1.6 - 3.5	100	73 - 221	1.1 - 3.4
	1 - 5y	101	93 - 213	1.4 - 3.3	115	126 - 216	1.9 - 3.4
	6 - 10y	99	104 - 198	1.6 - 3.0	99	110 - 195	1.7 - 3.0
	11 - 15y	97	88 - 176	1.3 - 2.7	100	104 - 184	1.6 - 2.9
	16 - 18y	100	86 - 178	1.3 - 2.8	104	101 - 151	1.5 - 2.4

Specimen Type: 1,2,3 Plasma, Serum

Reference:

1. Soldin SJ, Morales A, Albalos F, et al. Pediatric reference ranges on the Abbott IMx for FSH, LH, prolactin, TSH, T₄, T₃, free T₄, free T₃, T-uptake, IgE, and ferritin. Clin Biochem 1995;28:603-6.

2. Soldin SJ, Hicks JM, Bailey J, et al. Pediatric reference ranges for triiodothyronine. Clin Chem 1997;43:S199. (Abstract)

3. Murthy JN, Hicks JM, Soldin SJ. Evaluation of the Technicon Immuno I Random Access Immunoassay Analyzer and calculation of pediatric reference ranges for endocrine tests, T-uptake, and ferritin. Clin Biochem 1995;28:181-5.

Method(s):

1. Abbott IMx Analyzer. (Abbott Diagnostics, Inc., Abbott Park, IL.)

2. T₃ (Diagnostic Products, Inc. Los Angeles, CA).

3. Immuno I (Bayer Corp., Tarrytown NY)

Comments: 1,2,3 Study used hospitalized patients and a computerized approach adapted from the Hoffmann technique. Values are 2.5 - 97.5th percentiles.

TRIIODOTHYRONINE, FREE (FREE T₃)

Test	Age	Male			Female		
		n	ng/dL	pmol/L	n	ng/dL	pmol/L
1.	1 - 3d	24	0.14 - 0.48	2.2 - 7.4	26	0.14 - 0.54	2.2 - 8.3
	4 - 30d	73	0.14 - 0.55	2.2 - 8.4	62	0.15 - 0.50	2.3 - 7.7
	1 - 12mo	52	0.20 - 0.69	3.1 - 10.6	52	0.25 - 0.65	3.8 - 10.0
	1 - 5y	100	0.24 - 0.67	3.7 - 10.3	99	0.30 - 0.60	4.6 - 9.2
	6 - 10y	104	0.29 - 0.60	4.4 - 9.2	101	0.27 - 0.62	4.1 - 9.5
	11 - 15y	102	0.31 - 0.59	4.8 - 9.1	102	0.26 - 0.57	4.0 - 8.8
	16 - 18y	101	0.35 - 0.57	5.4 - 8.8	98	0.28 - 0.52	4.3 - 8.0
2.	0 - 6y	62	0.40 - 0.71	6.1 - 10.9	62	0.40 - 0.71	6.1 - 10.9
	7 - 12y	43	0.33 - 0.80	5.1 - 12.3	43	0.33 - 0.80	5.1 - 12.3
	13 - 18y	33	0.23 - 0.75	3.5 - 11.5	33	0.23 - 0.75	3.5 - 11.5

Specimen Type:	1,2	Plasma, Serum
Reference:	1.	Soldin SJ, Morales A, Albalos F, et al. Pediatric reference ranges on the Abbott IMx for FSH, LH, prolactin, TSH, T₄, T₃, free T₄, free T₃, T-uptake, IgE, and ferritin. Clin Biochem 1995;28:603-6.
	2.	Butler J, Moore P, Mieli-Vergani G, et al. Serum free thyroxine and free tri-iodothyronine in normal children. Ann Clin Biochem 1988;25:536-9.
Method(s):	1.	Abbott IMx Analyzer. (Abbott Diagnostics, Inc., Abbott Park, IL.)
	2.	RIA Amerlex (Amersham International plc, Cardiff, UK).
Comments:	1.	Study used hospitalized patients and a computerized approach adapted from the Hoffmann technique. Values are 2.5 - 97.5th percentiles.
	2.	Normal school children were used in this study. Data were log-transformed and the mean and standard deviation were calculated.

TRIIODOTHYRONINE UPTAKE TEST
(T₃U)

Test	Age	Male n	Male %	Female n	Female %
1.	1 - 365d	96	23 - 34	95	23 - 36
	1 - 3y	147	24 - 35	127	24 - 36
	4 - 6y	124	24 - 34	116	24 - 35
	7 - 12y	127	24 - 33	136	22 - 35
	13 - 15y	142	25 - 37	111	23 - 37
	16 - 18y	47	24 - 38	114	23 - 35

Test	Age	Male n	Male T-Uptake Units	Female n	Female T-Uptake Units
2.	1 - 30d	34	0.26 - 1.66	44	0.41 - 1.44
	1mo - 5y	99	0.72 - 1.35	141	0.81 - 1.36
	6 - 10y	96	0.74 - 1.22	98	0.78 - 1.18
	11 - 19y	113	0.58 - 1.23	108	0.76 - 1.25

Test	Age	Male n	Male Ratio	Female n	Female Ratio
3.	0 - 1mo	34	0.71 - 1.25	44	0.88 - 1.08
	1mo - 5y	99	0.89 - 1.13	141	0.92 - 1.13
	6 - 10y	96	0.84 - 1.08	98	0.82 - 1.10
	11 - 18y	113	0.88 - 1.08	108	0.77 - 1.16

Specimen Type:	1,2,3 Plasma, Serum
Reference:	1. Soldin SJ, Cook J, Beatey J, et al. Pediatric reference ranges for thyroxine and triiodothyronine. Clin Chem 1992;38:960. (Abstract)
	2. Soldin SJ, Morales A, Albalos F, et al. Pediatric reference ranges on the Abbott IMx for FSH, LH, prolactin, TSH, T₄, T₃, free T₄, free T₃, T-uptake, IgE, and ferritin. Clin Biochem 1995;28:603-6.
	3. Murthy JN, Hicks JM, Soldin SJ. Evaluation of the Technicon Immuno I Random Access Immunoassay Analyzer and calculation of pediatric reference ranges for endocrine tests, T-uptake, and ferritin. Clin Biochem 1995;28:181-5.
Method(s):	1. RIA Quantimmune® 11 (Bio-Rad, Bio-Rad Laboratories, Richmond, CA).
	2. Abbott IMx (Abbott Laboratories, Abbott Park, IL).
	3. Immuno I (Bayer Corp., Tarrytown, NY).
Comments:	1,2,3 Study used hospitalized patients and a computerized approach adapted from the Hoffmann technique to obtain the 2.5 - 97.5th percentiles.

TROPONIN I

Test	Age	Male and Female	
		n	97.5[th] percentile µg/L
1.	0 – 30d	97	4.8
	31 – 90d	46	0.4
	3 – 6mo	91	0.3
	7 – 12mo	53	0.2
	1 – 18y	57	<0.1

Specimen Type:	1	Serum/Plasma
Reference:	1.	Soldin SJ, Murthy JN, Agarwalla PK, et al. Pediatric Reference Ranges for Creatine Kinase, CKMB, Troponin I, and Cortisol. Clin Biochem 1999;32:77-80.
Method(s):	1.	Bayer Immuno I with Bayer Reagents (Bayer Corp., Tarrytown, NY)
Comments:	1.	Studies used hospitalized patients and a computerized approach to removing outliers adapted from the Hoffmann technic. Values are the 97.5[th] percentiles.

UREA NITROGEN

Test	Age		Male			Female	
		n	mg/dL	mmol/L	n	mg/dL	mmol/L
1.	1 - 7d	171	2 - 13	0.7 - 4.6	114	2 - 13	0.7 - 4.6
	8 - 30d	209	2 - 16	0.7 - 5.7	154	2 - 15	0.7 - 5.4
	1 - 3mo	278	2 - 12	0.7 - 4.3	274	2 - 14	0.7 - 5.0
	4 - 6mo	144	1 - 14	0.4 - 5.0	139	1 - 13	0.4 - 4.6
	7 - 12mo	204	2 - 14	0.7 - 5.0	160	1 - 13	0.4 - 4.6
2.	1 - 30d	51	4 - 12	1.4 - 4.3	43	3 - 17	1.1 - 6.1
	1 - 12mo	69	2 - 13	0.7 - 4.6	60	4 - 14	1.4 - 5.0
	1 - 3y	104	3 - 12	1.1 - 4.3	127	3 - 14	1.1 - 5.0
	4 - 6y	140	3 - 16	1.1 - 5.7	122	4 - 14	1.4 - 5.0
	7 - 9y	124	4 - 16	1.4 - 5.7	121	4 - 16	1.4 - 5.7
	10 - 12y	133	5 - 18	1.8 - 6.4	125	5 - 16	1.8 - 5.7
	13 - 15y	141	7 - 18	2.5 - 6.4	153	4 - 15	1.4 - 5.4
	16 - 18y	111	5 - 20	1.8 - 7.1	120	4 - 15	1.4 - 5.4

Test	Age		Male and Female		
			mg/dL	mmol/L	
3.	1 - 3y	50	5 - 17	1.8 - 6.0	
	4 - 6y	38	7 - 17	2.5 - 6.0	
	7 - 9y	72	7 - 17	2.5 - 6.0	
	10 - 11y	62	7 - 17	2.5 - 6.0	
	12 - 13y	73	7 - 17	2.5 - 6.0	
	14 - 15y	91	8 - 21	2.9 - 7.5	
	16 - 19y	107	8 - 21	2.9 - 7.5	

Specimen Type:	1, 2	Serum, Plasma
	3.	Plasma
Reference:	1.	Soldin SJ, Savwoir TV, Guo Y. Pediatric reference ranges for gamma-glutamyltransferase and urea nitrogen during the first year of life on the Vitros 500 analyzer. Clin Chem 1997;43:S199. (Abstract)
	2.	Soldin SJ, Bailey J, Beatey J, et al. Pediatric reference ranges for blood urea nitrogen (BUN) on the Hitachi 747 analyzer. Clin Chem 1996;42:S307. (Abstract)
	3.	Lockitch G, Halsted AC, Albersheim S, et al. Age and sex specific pediatric reference intervals for biochemistry analytes as measured with the Ektachem 700 analyzer. Clin Chem 1988;34:1622-5. (Abstract)
Method(s):	1, 3	Urease method, Ektachem 500 & 700 (Johnson & Johnson, Rochester, NY)
	2.	Hitachi 747 with Boehringer Mannheim reagents (Boehringer-Mannheim Diagnostics, Indianapolis, IN).
Comments:	1, 2	Study used hospitalized patients and a computerized approach adapted from the Hoffmann technique to obtain 2.5 - 97.5th percentiles.
	3.	Study used normal healthy children. Values are 2.5 - 97th percentiles.

URIC ACID

Test	Age	Male n	Male mg/dL	Male µmol/L	Female n	Female mg/dL	Female µmol/L
1.	1 - 30d	72	1.3 - 4.9	80 - 290	47	1.4 - 6.2	80 - 370
	1 - 3mo	83	1.4 - 5.3	80 - 310	64	1.4 - 5.8	80 - 340
	4 - 6mo	104	1.5 - 6.3	90 - 370	52	1.4 - 6.2	80 - 370
	7 - 12mo	97	1.5 - 6.6	90 - 390	65	1.5 - 6.2	90 - 370
2.	1 - 3y	49*	1.8 - 5.0	105 - 300	49*	1.8 - 5.0	105 - 300
	4 - 6y	38*	2.2 - 4.7	130 - 280	38*	2.2 - 4.7	130 - 280
	7 - 9y	72*	2.0 - 5.0	120 - 295	72*	2.0 - 5.0	120 - 295
	10 - 11y	28	2.3 - 5.4	135 - 320	34	3.0 - 4.7	180 - 280
	12 - 13y	32	2.7 - 6.7	160 - 400	40	3.0 - 5.8	180 - 345
	14 - 15y	39	2.4 - 7.8	140 - 465	50	3.0 - 5.8	180 - 345
	16 - 19y	41	4.0 - 8.6	235 - 510	68	3.0 - 5.9	180 - 350
3.	1 - 30d	84	1.2 - 3.9	71 - 230	91	1.0 - 4.6	59 - 271
	31 - 365d	138	1.2 - 5.6	71 - 330	110	1.1 - 5.4	65 - 319
	1 - 3y	149	2.1 - 5.6	124 - 330	105	1.8 - 5.0	106 - 295
	4 - 6y	120	1.8 - 5.5	106 - 325	91	2.0 - 5.1	118 - 301
	7 - 9y	123	1.8 - 5.4	106 - 319	115	1.8 - 5.5	106 - 325
	10 - 12y	121	2.2 - 5.8	130 - 342	92	2.5 - 5.9	148 - 348
	13 - 15y	106	3.1 - 7.0	183 - 413	116	2.2 - 6.4	130 - 378
	16 - 18y	82	2.1 - 7.6	124 - 448	111	2.4 - 6.6	142 - 389

Specimen Type:

1, 3   Plasma, Serum
2.   Serum

Reference:

1. Soldin SJ, Savwoir TV, Guo Y. Pediatric reference ranges for lactate dehydrogenase and uric acid during the first year of life on the Vitros 500 analyzer. Clin Chem 1997;43:S199. (Abstract)

2. Lockitch G, Halstead AC, Albersheim S, et al. Age and sex specific pediatric reference intervals for biochemistry analytes as measured with the Ektachem 700 analyzer. Clin Chem 1988;34:1622-5.

3. Soldin SJ, Bailey J, Beatey J, et al. Pediatric reference ranges for uric acid. Clin Chem 1996;42:S308. (Abstract)

Method(s):

1,2 Uricase on Kodak Ektachem analyzer (Johnson & Johnson, Rochester, NY).

3. Hitachi 747 analyzer with Boehringer Mannheim reagents (Boehringer-Mannheim Diagnostics, Indianapolis, IN).

Comments:

1,3 Study used hospitalized patients and a computerized approach adapted from the Hoffmann technique to obtain the 2.5 - 97.5th percentiles.

2. Study performed on healthy children. Results are 2.5 - 97.5th percentiles.

*No significant differences were found for males and females.
These ranges were therefore derived from combined data.

URINE VOLUME (24h)		
	Male and Female	
Age	**mL**	**L**
Newborn	50 - 300	0.05 - 0.30
Infant	350 - 550	0.35 - 0.55
Child	500 - 1000	0.50 - 1.00
Adolescent	700 - 1400	0.70 - 1.40
Thereafter	600 - 1800	0.60 - 1.80

Specimen Type:	Urine (24h)
Reference:	Behrman RE, Ed. Nelson textbook of pediatrics, 14th ed. Philadelphia, PA: WB Saunders Company, 1992:1824.
Method(s):	Not given.
Comments:	Varies with intake and other factors.

VANILLYLMANDELIC ACID (VMA) (URINE)
4-HYDROXY-3-METHOXYMANDELIC ACID

Test	Age	n	mg/g creatinine	mmol/ mol creatinine	n	mg/24h	μmol/24h
			Male and Female				
1.	0 - 1y	37	< 18.8	< 10.7	48	< 2.3	< 11.6
	2 - 4y	49	< 11.0	< 6.3	34	< 3.0	< 15.1
	5 - 9y	79	< 8.3	< 4.7	20	< 3.5	< 17.7
	10 - 19y	55	< 8.2	< 4.7	40	< 6.0	< 30.3
	> 19y	56	< 6.0	< 3.4	56	< 6.8	< 34.3
2.	0 - 3mo	12	5.9 - 37.0	3.4 - 21.1			
	3 - 12mo	28	8.4 - 43.8	4.8 - 25.0			
	1 - 2y	15	7.9 - 23.0	4.5 - 13.1			
	2 - 5y	22	2.9 - 23.0	1.7 - 13.1			
	5 - 10y	21	5.8 - 18.7	3.3 - 10.7			
	10 - 15y	13	1.6 - 10.6	0.9 - 6.1			
	> 15y	8	2.8 - 8.3	1.6 - 4.7			

Specimen Type: 1,2   Urine

Reference:
1. Soldin SJ, Hill JG. Liquid chromatographic analysis for urinary 4-hydroxy-3-methoxy-mandelic acid and 4-hydroxy-3-methoxyphenyl acetic acid and its use in investigation of neural crest tumors. Clin Chem 1981;27:502-3.

2. Tuchman M, Morris CL, Ramnaraine ML, et al. Value of random urinary homovanillic acid and vanillylmandelic acid levels in the diagnosis and management of patients with neuroblastoma: comparison with 24-hour urine collections. Pediatrics 1985;75:324-8.

Method(s):
1. HPLC with electrochemical detection.
2. Capillary gas chromatography.

Comments:
1. Analysis performed on patients under investigation of hypertension or not suspected of having a neural crest tumor. All patients studied free of neoplasia. Results are 95th percentile.

2. Values are 0 - 100th percentiles. Normal values were obtained from 93 pediatric patients in whom the diagnosis of neural crest tumors had been excluded.

VITAMIN A
(RETINOL)

Test	Age	Male and Female		
		n	µmol/L	µg/dL
1.	At Birth	25	0.49 - 1.81	14 - 52
	Adult (mothers)	25	0.71 - 2.27	20 - 65
2.	1 - 6y	62*	0.7 - 1.5	20 - 43
	7 - 12y	23*	0.9 - 1.7	20 - 49
	13 - 19y	24*	0.9 - 2.5	26 - 72
3.	Term Neonates (> 37 weeks)	41	0.63 - 1.75	18 - 50
	Preterm Neonates (< 36.6 weeks)	58	0.46 - 1.61	13 - 46

Specimen Type:	1,2	Serum
	3.	Serum, Plasma
Reference:	1.	Jansson L, Nilsson B. Serum retinol and retinol-binding protein in mothers and infants at delivery. Biol Neonate 1983;43:269-71.
	2.	Lockitch G, Halstead A, Wadsworth L, et al. Age and sex specific pediatric reference intervals for zinc, copper, selenium, iron, vitamins A and E and related proteins. Clin Chem 1988;34:1625-8.
	3.	Cardona-Pérez A, et al. Cord blood retinol and retinol binding protein in preterm and term neonates. Nutrition Research 1996:16;191-6.
Method(s):	1.	Affinity chromatography and HPLC. See reference.
	2,3	HPLC. See reference for description.
Comments:	1.	Results are mean ± 2SD. Retinol studied in 25 healthy newborns and their mothers.
	2.	The study population was healthy children. Non-parametric methods were used to determine the 0.025 and 0.975 fractiles.
		*No significant differences were found for males and females. These ranges were therefore derived from combined data.
	3.	Healthy term and preterm neonates studied. Results are 2.5 - 97.5th percentiles.

VITAMIN B$_{12}$

Test	Age	Male n	Male pmol/L	Female n	Female pmol/L
1.	0 - 1y	127	216 - 891	94	168 - 1117
	2 - 3y	142	195 - 897	133	307 - 392
	4 - 6y	156	181 - 795	111	231 - 1038
	7 - 9y	103	200 - 863	103	182 - 866
	10 - 12y	105	135 - 803	94	145 - 752
	13 - 18y	159	158 - 638	159	134 - 605
2.	Newborn[a]	*	130 - 590	*	130 - 590
	After newborn period[a]	*	100 - 520	*	100 - 520
	Adult[b]	*	120 - 700	*	120 - 700

Specimen Type:
1. Plasma
2. Serum

Reference:
1. Hicks JM, Cook J, Godwin ID, et al. Vitamin B$_{12}$ and folate: Pediatric reference ranges. Arch Pathol Lab Med 1993;117:704-6.

2. a. Behrman RE, Vaughan VC, Eds. Nelson textbook of pediatrics. Philadelphia, PA: WB Saunders 1983:1827-60.
   b. Hall CA, Bardwell SA, Allen ES, et al. Variation in plasma folate levels among groups of healthy persons. Am J Clin Nutr, 1975;28:854-7.

Method(s):
1. Radioimmunoassay Quantaphase B$_{12}$ (BioRad, Hercules, CA).
2. See references for particulars of assays used.

Comments:
1. Study used hospitalized patients and a computerized approach adapted from the Hoffmann technique. Values are 2.5 - 97.5th percentiles.

2. *Numbers not available.

184

25-HYDROXY VITAMIN D (25 OH VIT D)

Test	Age	Male				Female			
		Summer		Winter		Summer		Winter	
		n	μg/L	n	μg/L	n	μg/L	n	μg/L
1.	1 - 30d	61	6.2 - 33.4	46	3.3 - 28.8	62	6.4 - 30.7	34	1.9 - 32.0
	31 - 365d	76	18.6 - 36.9	71	7.4 - 53.3	87	16.0 - 48.2	64	11.6 - 36.7
	1 - 3y	144	6.9 - 46.8	90	10.1 - 39.0	129	11.6 - 48.9	109	11.3 - 41.1
	4 - 12y	171	4.6 - 37.4	151	6.3 - 36.0	161	2.8 - 36.7	59	8.4 - 29.9
	13 - 18y	121	4.3 - 31.4	41	2.0 - 29.1	130	2.3 - 28.3	63	1.8 - 20.4
2.	1 - 30d	61	11 – 44	46	8 – 38	62	11 – 41	34	6 – 42
	1mo – <1y	76	26 – 48	71	13 – 68	87	23 – 62	64	18 – 48
	1 - 3y	144	12 – 60	90	16 – 51	129	18 – 62	109	17 – 53
	4 - 12y	171	9 – 49	151	11 - 47	161	7 – 48	59	14 – 40
	13 - 18y	121	9 - 41	41	6 - 39	130	7 - 38	63	6 - 28

Specimen Type:	1,2. Serum
Reference:	1. Soldin SJ, Hicks JM, Bailey J, et al. Pediatric reference ranges for 25 hydroxy vitamin D during the summer and winter. Clin Chem 1997;43:S200. (Abstract)
	2. Soldin SJ, Murthy J, Lauber B, et al. Pediatric Reference Ranges for 25-Hydroxy Vitamin D using DiaSorin Kit. Clin Chem 1998;44;A14 (Abstract).
Method(s):	1. Radioimmunoassay. Nichols Institute Diagnostics Kit (Nichols Institue Diagnostics, Capistrano, CA)
	2. Radioimmunoassay, Diasorin Kit, Diasorin, Stillwater, MN.
Comments:	1,2. Study used hospitalized patients and a computerized approach adapted from the Hoffmann technique. Values are the 2.5 - 97.5th percentiles.

VITAMIN E
(α-TOCOPHEROL)

Test	Age	n	Male and Female	
			μmol/L	μg/mL
1.	1 - 6y	62*	7 - 21	3.0 - 9.0
	7 - 12y	23*	10 - 21	4.0 - 9.0
	13 - 19y	24*	13 - 24	6.0 - 10.1
2.	Prematures	**	1 - 8	0.5 - 3.5
	Full Term	**	2 - 8	1.0 - 3.5
	2 - 5mo	**	5 - 14	2.0 - 6.0
	6 - 24mo	**	8 - 19	3.5 - 8.0
	2 - 12y	**	13 - 21	5.5 - 9.0

Specimen Type:	1. Serum 2. Plasma, Serum
Reference:	1. Lockitch G, Halstead A, Wadsworth L, et al. Age and sex specific pediatric reference intervals for zinc, copper, selenium, iron, vitamins A and E and related proteins. Clin Chem 1988;34:1625-8. 2. Meites S, Ed. Pediatric clinical chemistry, 3rd ed. Washington, DC: AACC Press, 1989:295-6.
Method(s):	1. HPLC. 2. Hansen LG, Warwick WJ. An improved assay method for vitamins A and E using fluorometry. Am J Clin Path 1978;70:922-3. McWhirter WR. Plasma tocopherol in infants and children. Acta Path Scand 1975:64;446-8.
Comments:	1. The study population was healthy children. Non-parametric methods were used to determine the 0.025 and 0.975 fractiles. *No significant differences were found for males and females. These ranges were therefore derived from combined data. 2. **See references for numbers used in study.

ZINC

Test	Age	n	μg/dL	μmol/L	n	μg/dL	μmol/L
		Male			**Female**		
1.	0 - 5d	27*	65 - 140	9.9 - 21.4	27*	65 - 140	9.9 - 21.4
	1 - 5y	77*	67 - 118	10.3 - 18.1	77*	67 - 118	10.3 - 18.1
	6 - 9y	44*	77 - 107	11.8 - 16.4	44*	77 - 107	11.8 - 16.4
	10 - 14y	36	76 - 101	11.6 - 15.4	23	79 - 118	12.1 - 18.0
	15 - 19y	55	64 - 104	9.8 - 15.4	31	60 - 101	9.2 - 15.4
2.	3 - 5y	38**	71 - 149	10.9 - 22.8	38**	71 - 149	10.9 - 22.8
	6 - 8y	43**	70 - 128	10.7 - 19.6	43**	70 - 128	10.7 - 19.6
	9 - 11y	52**	64 - 124	9.8 - 19.0	52**	64 - 124	9.8 - 19.0
	12 - 13y	24**	45 - 125	6.9 - 19.1	24**	45 - 125	6.9 - 19.1
	14 - 16y	29**	42 - 125	6.4 - 19.1	29**	42 - 125	6.4 - 19.1
3.			**Male and Female**				
			μg/dL		μmol/L		
	0 - <0.5y	13	26 – 141		4.0 – 21.6		
	0.5 - <1.0y	18	29 – 131		4.5 – 20.1		
	1.0 - <2.0y	15	31 – 120		4.8 – 18.4		
	2.0 - <4.0y	23	29 – 115		4.4 – 17.6		
	4.0 - <6.0y	19	48 – 119		7.4 – 18.2		
	6.0 - <10.0y	25	48 – 129		7.3 – 19.7		
	10.0 - <14.0y	21	25 – 148		3.9 – 22.7		
	14.0 - <18.0y	17	46 – 130		7.1 – 19.9		

Specimen Type:	1,2. Serum 3. Serum/Plasma
Reference:	1. Lockitch G, Halstead A, Wadsworth L, et al. Age and sex specific pediatric reference intervals for zinc, copper, selenium, iron, vitamins A and E and related proteins. Clin Chem 1988;34:1625-8. 2. Malvy DJ-M, Arnaud J, Burtschy, B, et al. Reference values for serum, zinc and selenium of French healthy children. Eur J Epidemiol 1993;9:155-61 3. Rükgauer M, Klein J, Kruse-Jarres JD. Reference Values for the Trace Elements Copper, Manganese, Selenium, and Zinc in the Serum/Plasma of Children, Adolescents and Adults. J. Trace Elements Med. Biol. 1997;11:92-8.
Method(s):	1. Atomic absorption spectrometry with deuterium background correction Varian AA-1475 (Varian Canada, Inc., Georgetown, Canada). 2. Perkin Elmer Atomic Absorption Spectrophotometry (Perkin-Elmer Corporation, Rockville, MD). 3. Atomic Absorption Spectrophotometry with Zeeman background compensation. Perkin Elmer ETAAS, Zeeman 3030, Uberlingen, Germany.
Comments:	1. The study population was healthy children. Non-parametric methods were used to determine the 0.025 and 0.975 fractiles. *No significant differences were found for males and females. These ranges were therefore derived from combined data. 2. The study population consisted of healthy French children. Values reported are the 2.5 - 97.5th percentiles. **No significant differences were found for males and females. These ranges were therefore derived from combined data. 3. Study population was drawn from patients visiting the outpatient department or surgical or orthopedic ward for preoperative work up. Results are mean ± 2 S.D.s (2.5th – 97.5th percentiles).

Hematology Tests

Hematology Test

ATYPICAL LYMPHOCYTE COUNT (RELATIVE)

Test	Age	Male		Female	
		n	%	n	%
1.	1 - 14d	35	4.6 - 10.3	27	3.3 - 10.7
	15 - 30d	33	3.9 - 12.2	27	3.9 - 9.7
	31 - 60d	146	4.6 - 10.1	108	4.0 - 7.9
	61 - 180d	458	3.7 - 10.2	3449	3.7 - 9.2
	0.5 - <2y	1524	3.4 - 8.7	1229	3.4 - 9.5
	2 - <6y	1600	2.6 - 7.3	1276	2.6 - 7.4
	6 - <12y	1453	2.1 - 5.6	1369	2.1 - 5.7
	12 - <18y	1375	1.9 - 5.3	1729	1.9 - 4.9
	>18y	688	1.8 - 5.0	1058	1.8 - 4.6

Specimen Type:	1. Whole blood (K$_2$/EDTA anticoagulant)
Reference:	1. Brugnara C. Manuscript in preparation.
Method(s):	1. Bayer ADVIA 120 (Bayer Diagnostics, Tarrytown, NY)
Comments:	1. Data from outpatients. A computerized approach adapted from the Hoffmann technique was utilized to remove outliers and obtain the 2.5th and 97.5th percentiles.

191

BASOPHIL COUNT (RELATIVE)

Test	Age	Male n	Male %	Male Number Fraction	Female n	Female %	Female Number Fraction
1.	1 - 3d	48	0 - 2.3	0 - .023	50	0 - 2.1	0 - .021
	4 - 7d	33	0 - 2.4	0 - .024	29	0 - 2.7	0 - .027
	8 - 14d	43	0 - 1.8	0 - .018	58	0 - 1.8	0 - .018
	15 - 30d	137	0 - 1.2	0 - .012	98	0 - 1.1	0 - .011
	31 - 60d	462	0 - 1.0	0 - .010	359	0 - 0.9	0 - .009
	61 - 180d	1472	0 - 1.0	0 - .010	1165	0 - 1.0	0 - .010
	0.5 - <2y	5932	0 - 1.0	0 - .010	4606	0 - 1.1	0 - .011
	2 - <6y	6573	0 - 1.0	0 - .010	5671	0 - 1.0	0 - .010
	6 - <12y	5347	0 - 1.0	0 - .010	4723	0 - 1.1	0 - .011
	12 - <18y	3955	0 - 1.1	0 - .011	5111	0 - 1.0	0 - .010
	> 18y	1968	0 - 1.2	0 - .012	3055	0 - 1.0	0 - .010
2.	1 - 14d	35	0 - 1.8	0 - .018	28	0 - 2.1	0 - .021
	15 - 30d	37	0 - 0.8	0 - .008	32	0 - 1.1	0 - .011
	31 - 60d	151	0 - 0.9	0 - .009	117	0 - 1.3	0 - .013
	61 - 180d	474	0 - 1.1	0 - .011	365	0 - 1.1	0 - .011
	0.5 - <2y	1570	0 - 1.0	0 - .010	1262	0 - 1.1	0 - .011
	2 - <6y	1635	0 - 0.9	0 - .009	1310	0 - 0.9	0 - .009
	6 - <12y	1467	0 - 0.8	0 - .008	1391	0 - 0.9	0 - .009
	12 - <18y	1391	0 - 0.8	0 - .008	1755	0 - 0.8	0 - .008
	>18y	691	0 - 0.9	0 - .009	1066	0 - 0.8	0 - .008

Specimen Type:	1. Whole blood (K$_3$/EDTA anticoagulant) 2. Whole blood (K$_2$/EDTA anticoagulant)
Reference:	1. Pediatric Reference Ranges, Eds. Soldin SJ, Brugnara C, et. al. 2nd Edition 1997 AACC Press. 2. Brugnara C. Manuscript in preparation.
Method(s):	1. Bayer H*3 (Bayer Diagnostics, Tarrytown, NY) 2. Bayer ADVIA 120 (Bayer Diagnostics, Tarrytown, NY)
Comments:	1,2. Data from outpatients. A computerized approach adapted from the Hoffmann technique was utilized to remove outliers and obtain the 2.5th and 97.5th percentiles.

RETICULOCYTE CELLULAR HEMOGLOBIN
CONTENT (CHR)

Test	Age	Male		Female	
		n	pg/cell	n	pg/cell
1.	1d - <2y	132	22.5 - 31.8	104	23.9 - 30.9
	2 - <6y	127	25.1 - 32.0	92	26.4 - 32.1
	6 - <12y	133	23.6 - 33.9	116	25.1 - 33.3
	12 - <18y	211	27.0 - 33.2	221	28.2 - 33.9
	>18y	214	30.1 - 34.6	402	27.1 - 35.2

Specimen Type:	1.	Whole blood (K$_2$/EDTA anticoagulant)
Reference:	1.	Brugnara C. Manuscript in preparation.
Method(s):	1.	Bayer ADVIA 120 (Bayer Diagnostics, Tarrytown, NY)
Comments:	1.	Data from outpatients. A computerized approach adapted from the Hoffmann technique was utilized to remove outliers and obtain the 2.5th and 97.5th percentiles.

EOSINOPHIL COUNT (ABSOLUTE)

Test	Age	Male n	Male × 10³/µL	Male × 10⁹/L	Female n	Female × 10³/µL	Female × 10⁹/L
1.	1 - 3d	41	0 - 0.6	0 - 0.6	43	0 - 0.6	0 - 0.6
	4 - 7d	26	0 - 0.7	0 - 0.7	25	0 - 0.6	0 - 0.6
	8 - 14d	39	0 - 0.8	0 - 0.8	52	0 - 0.6	0 - 0.6
	15 - 30d	125	0 - 0.8	0 - 0.8	85	0 - 0.7	0 - 0.7
	31 - 60d	381	0 - 0.6	0 - 0.6	284	0 - 0.5	0 - 0.5
	61 - 180d	1214	0 - 0.5	0 - 0.5	953	0 - 0.4	0 - 0.4
	0.5 - <2y	4935	0 - 0.3	0 - 0.3	3820	0 - 0.3	0 - 0.3
	2 - <6y	5641	0 - 0.3	0 - 0.3	4856	0 - 0.3	0 - 0.3
	6 - <12y	4690	0 - 0.4	0 - 0.4	4146	0 - 0.3	0 - 0.3
	12 - <18y	3515	0 - 0.4	0 - 0.4	4530	0 - 0.3	0 - 0.3
	≥ 18y	1762	0 - 0.3	0 - 0.3	2744	0 - 0.3	0 - 0.3
2.	1 - 3d	172	0 - 0.3	0 - 0.3	114	0 - 0.2	0 - 0.2
	4 - 7d	152	0 - 0.8	0 - 0.8	108	0 - 0.5	0 - 0.5
	8 - 14d	180	0 - 0.6	0 - 0.6	124	0 - 0.6	0 - 0.6
	15 - 30d	390	0 - 0.9	0 - 0.9	291	0 - 0.5	0 - 0.5
	31 - 60d	74	0 - 0.5	0 - 0.5	184	0 - 0.2	0 - 0.2
	61 - 180d	75	0 - 0.4	0 - 0.4	102	0 - 0.1	0 - 0.1
	0.5 - <2y	177	0 - 0.3	0 - 0.3	119	0 - 0.2	0 - 0.2
	2 - <6y	189	0 - 0.2	0 - 0.2	134	0 - 0.2	0 - 0.2
	6 - <12y	126	0 - 0.3	0 - 0.3	136	0 - 0.2	0 - 0.2
	12 - 18y	140	0 - 0.3	0 - 0.3	154	0 - 0.2	0 - 0.2
3.	1 - 14d	38	0 - 0.7	0 - 0.7	28	0 - 0.6	0 - 0.6
	15 - 30d	35	0 - 0.9	0 - 0.9	27	0 - 0.4	0 - 0.4
	31 - 60d	146	0 - 0.6	0 - 0.6	109	0 - 0.5	0 - 0.5
	61 - 180d	471	0 - 0.4	0 - 0.4	359	0 - 0.4	0 - 0.4
	0.5 - <2y	1558	0 - 0.4	0 - 0.4	1257	0 - 0.3	0 - 0.3
	2 - <6y	1646	0 - 0.4	0 - 0.4	1331	0 - 0.3	0 - 0.3
	6 - <12y	1600	0 - 0.5	0 - 0.5	1411	0 - 0.3	0 - 0.3
	12 - <18y	1430	0 - 0.3	0 - 0.3	1799	0 - 0.3	0 - 0.3
	>18y	717	0 - 0.4	0 - 0.4	1092	0 - 0.3	0 - 0.3

Specimen Type:	1,2.	Whole blood (K_3/EDTA anticoagulant)
	3.	Whole blood (K_2/EDTA anticoagulant)
Reference:	1, 2	Pediatric Reference Ranges, Eds. Soldin SJ, Brugnara C, et. al. 2nd Edition 1997 AACC Press.
	3.	Brugnara C. Manuscript in preparation.
Method(s):	1.	Bayer H*3 (Bayer Diagnostics, Tarrytown, NY)
	2.	Coulter STKS (Beckman Coulter Inc., Brea, CA)
	3.	Bayer ADVIA 120 (Bayer Diagnostics, Tarrytown, NY)
Comments:	1,3.	Data from outpatients. A computerized approach adapted from the Hoffmann technique was utilized to remove outliers and obtain the 2.5th and 97.5th percentiles.
	2.	Data from hospitalized patients (excluding hematology, oncology, and intensive care unit patients). A computerized approach adapted from the Hoffmann technique was utilized to remove outliers and obtain the 2.5th and 97.5th percentiles.

EOSINOPHIL COUNT (RELATIVE)

Test	Age	Male n	%	Number Fraction	Female n	%	Number Fraction
1.	1 - 3d	55	0 - 8.0	0 - .080	54	0 - 5.6	0 - .056
	4 - 7d	35	0 - 5.9	0 - .059	31	0 - 5.1	0 - .051
	8 - 14d	44	0 - 6.7	0 - .067	61	0 - 5.6	0 - .056
	15 - 30d	148	0 - 6.4	0 - .064	104	0 - 5.1	0 - .051
	31 - 60d	487	0 - 5.7	0 - .057	374	0 - 4.7	0 - .047
	61 - 180d	1526	0 - 4.6	0 - .046	1200	0 - 3.7	0 - .037
	0.5 -<2y	6136	0 - 3.3	0 - .033	4741	0 - 2.7	0 - .027
	2 - <6y	6713	0 - 4.3	0 - .043	5811	0 - 3.4	0 - .034
	6 - <12y	5340	0 - 5.8	0 - .058	4812	0 - 4.7	0 - .047
	12 - <18y	4009	0 - 5.5	0 - .055	5199	0 - 3.9	0 - .039
	>18y	2014	0 - 5.3	0 - .053	3109	0 - 3.5	0 - .035
2.	1 - 3d	172	0 - 2.9	0 - .029	114	0 - 2.9	0 - .029
	4 - 7d	152	0 - 5.4	0 - .054	108	0 - 7.5	0 - .075
	8 - 14d	180	0 - 5.0	0 - .050	124	0 - 4.1	0 - .041
	15 - 30d	390	0 - 7.0	0 - .070	290	0 - 5.4	0 - .054
	31 - 60d	74	0 - 5.4	0 - .054	184	0 - 3.1	0 - .031
	61 - 180d	75	0 - 3.5	0 - .035	102	0 - 2.8	0 - .028
	0.5 - <2y	177	0 - 2.0	0 - .020	119	0 - 3.1	0 - .031
	2 - <6y	189	0 - 2.4	0 - .024	134	0 - 3.3	0 - .033
	6 - <12y	126	0 - 4.8	0 - .048	136	0 - 4.0	0 - .040
	12 - 18y	140	0 - 2.8	0 - .028	154	0 - 4.1	0 - .041
3.	1 - 14d	38	0 - 6.1	0 - .061	28	0 - 4.2	0 - .042
	15 - 30d	33	0 - 7.0	0 - .070	27	0 - 4.0	0 - .040
	31 - 60d	148	0 - 5.7	0 - .057	109	0 - 5.0	0 - .050
	61 - 180d	469	0 - 4.3	0 - .043	357	0 - 3.8	0 - .038
	0.5 - <2y	1555	0 - 3.5	0 - .035	1254	0 - 2.8	0 - .028
	2 - <6y	1636	0 - 4.2	0 - .042	1317	0 - 3.9	0 - .039
	6 - <12y	1487	0 - 5.6	0 - .056	1395	0 - 4.2	0 - .042
	12 - <18y	1413	0 - 4.5	0 - .045	1770	0 - 3.7	0 - .037
	>18y	713	0 - 4.9	0 - .049	1079	0 - 3.9	0 - .039

Specimen Type:	1,2. Whole blood (K_3/EDTA anticoagulant)
	3. Whole blood (K_2/EDTA anticoagulant)
Reference:	1, 2 Pediatric Reference Ranges, Eds. Soldin SJ, Brugnara C, et. al. 2nd Edition 1997 AACC Press.
	3. Brugnara C. Manuscript in preparation.
Method(s):	1. Bayer H*3 (Bayer Diagnostics, Tarrytown, NY)
	2. Coulter STKS (Beckman Coulter Inc., Brea, CA)
	3. Bayer ADVIA 120 (Bayer Diagnostics, Tarrytown, NY)
Comments:	1,3. Data from outpatients. A computerized approach adapted from the Hoffmann technique was utilized to remove outliers and obtain the 2.5th and 97.5th percentiles.
	2. Data from hospitalized patients (excluding hematology, oncology, and intensive care unit patients). A computerized approach adapted from the Hoffmann technique was utilized to remove outliers and obtain the 2.5th and 97.5th percentiles.

HEMATOCRIT

Test	Age	Male			Female		
		n	%	Volume Fraction	n	%	Volume Fraction
1.	1 - 3d	76	43.4 - 56.1	.434 - .561	76	37.4 - 55.9	.374 - .559
	4 - 7d	49	40.2 - 54.7	.402 - .547	39	39.1 - 56.7	.391 - .567
	8 - 14d	61	33.7 - 51.1	.337 - .511	69	36.4 - 51.2	.364 - .512
	15 - 30d	168	29.7 - 44.2	.297 - .442	116	30.6 - 44.7	.306 - .447
	31 - 60d	562	26.2 - 35.3	.262 - .353	419	26.3 - 36.6	.263 - .366
	61 - 180d	1842	28.7 - 36.1	.287 - .361	1364	28.5 - 36.1	.285 - .361
	0.5 - <2y	8859	30.9 - 37.0	.309 - .370	6993	31.2 - 37.2	.312 - .372
	2 - <6y	11146	31.7 - 37.7	.317 - .377	9750	32.0 - 37.1	.320 - .371
	6 - <12y	7468	32.7 - 39.3	.327 - .393	6799	33.0 - 39.6	.330 - .396
	12 - <18y	5551	34.8 - 43.9	.348 - .439	7995	34.0 - 40.7	.340 - .407
	> 18y	3175	33.4 - 46.2	.334 - .462	8608	33.0 - 41.0	.330 - .410
2.	1 - 3d	216	33.5 - 52.7	.335 - .527	143	38.4 - 56.0	.384 - .560
	4 - 7d	211	36.9 - 50.1	.369 - .501	132	34.4 - 50.8	.344 - .508
	8 - 14d	226	33.4 - 49.0	.334 - .490	151	32.9 - 47.5	.329 - .475
	15 - 30d	445	30.7 - 44.9	.307 - .449	338	31.9 - 45.2	.319 - .452
	31 - 60d	81	27.0 - 35.8	.270 - .358	197	27.1 - 41.9	.271 - .419
	61 - 180d	86	29.9 - 39.0	.299 - .390	109	28.6 - 42.3	.286 - .423
	0.5 - <2y	198	28.3 - 40.0	.283 - .400	139	28.1 - 39.1	.281 - .391
	2 - <6y	204	28.5[a] - 37.9	.285[a] - .379	147	32.0[a] - 39.8	.320[a] - .398
	6 - <12y	141	31.6[a] - 39.5	.316[a] - .395	148	32.0[a] - 40.0	.320[a] - .400
	12 - 18y	155	27.3[a] - 43.6	.273[a] - .436	172	27.9[a] - 39.6	.279[a] - .396
3.	1 - 14d	48	36.2 - 58.5	.362 - .585	35	39.1 - 58.5	.391 - .585
	15 - 30d	41	26.7 - 50.3	.267 - .503	34	31.8 - 46.9	.318 - .469
	31 - 60d	172	25.2 - 37.1	.252 - .371	130	27.2 - 41.6	.272 - .416
	61 - 180d	524	28.2 - 39.7	.282 - .397	389	28.8 - 39.5	.288 - .395
	0.5 - <2y	2041	30.8 - 39.1	.308 - .391	1689	30.7 - 39.3	.307 - .393
	2 - <6y	2386	31.5 - 40.4	.315 - .404	2022	31.6 - 40.4	.316 - .404
	6 - <12y	1919	32.0 - 41.9	.320 - .419	1786	32.0 - 41.8	.320 - .418
	12 - <18y	1738	32.3 - 46.8	.323 - .468	2408	33.1 - 43.4	.331 - .434
	>18y	1038	30.0 - 48.9	.300 - .489	2479	32.6 - 43.7	.326 - .437

Specimen Type:	1,2. Whole blood (K_3/EDTA anticoagulant)
	3. Whole blood (K_2/EDTA anticoagulant)
Reference:	1, 2 Pediatric Reference Ranges, Eds. Soldin SJ, Brugnara C, et. al. 2nd Edition 1997 AACC Press.
	3. Brugnara C. Manuscript in preparation.
Method(s):	1. Bayer H*3 (Bayer Diagnostics, Tarrytown, NY)
	2. Coulter STKS (Beckman Coulter Inc., Brea, CA)
	3. Bayer ADVIA 120 (Bayer Diagnostics, Tarrytown, NY)
Comments:	1,3. Data from outpatients. A computerized approach adapted from the Hoffmann technique was utilized to remove outliers and obtain the 2.5th and 97.5th percentiles (1). The upper 90% of the data was used for the Hoffman Plot for set 3.
	2. Data from hospitalized patients (excluding hematology, oncology, and intensive care unit patients). A computerized approach adapted from the Hoffmann technique was utilized to remove outliers and obtain the 2.5th and 97.5th percentiles.
	[a]To obtain the 2.5th percentile, the statistical technique was modified to use the central 60% of the data for the Hoffmann plot.

HEMOGLOBIN

Test	Age	Male			Female		
		n	g/dL	g/L	n	g/dL	g/L
1.	1 - 3d	76	14.7 - 18.6	147 - 186	76	12.7 - 18.3	127 - 183
	4 - 7d	49	13.4 - 17.9	134 - 179	38	12.2 - 18.7	122 - 187
	8 - 14d	61	11.1 - 16.7	111 - 167	69	11.9 - 16.9	119 - 169
	15 - 30d	168	9.9 - 14.9	99 - 149	116	10.5 - 14.7	105 - 147
	31 - 60d	562	8.9 - 11.9	89 - 119	419	8.9 - 12.3	89 - 123
	61 - 180d	1839	9.7 - 12.2	97 - 122	1361	9.7 - 12.0	97 - 120
	0.5 - <2y	8829	10.3 - 12.4	103 - 124	6917	10.4 - 12.4	104 - 124
	2 - <6y	11123	10.5 - 12.7	105 - 127	9729	10.7 - 12.7	107 - 127
	6 - <12y	7458	11.0 - 13.3	110 - 133	6778	10.9 - 13.3	109 - 133
	12 - <18y	5546	11.5 - 14.8	115 - 148	7989	11.2 - 13.6	112 - 136
	> 18y	3167	10.9 - 15.7	109 - 157	8600	10.7 - 13.5	107 - 135
2.	1 - 3d	217	12.2 - 17.9	122 - 179	144	13.2 - 18.4	132 - 184
	4 - 7d	209	12.8 - 16.9	128 - 169	132	11.8 - 17.7	118 - 177
	8 - 14d	224	11.8 - 16.8	118 - 168	151	11.5 - 16.3	115 - 163
	15 - 30d	447	10.6 - 15.4	106 - 154	339	10.9 - 15.3	109 - 153
	31 - 60d	82	9.0 - 12.1	90 - 121	197	9.2 - 14.4	92 - 144
	61 - 180d	98	10.0 - 13.2	100 - 132	123	9.8 - 13.7	98 - 137
	0.5 - <2y	199	9.8 - 13.4	98 - 134	143	9.6 - 13.1	96 - 131
	2 - <6y	200	9.6[a] - 12.8	96[a] - 128	144	10.9[a] - 13.4	109[a] - 134
	6 - <12y	135	10.7[a] - 13.5	107[a] - 135	143	10.9[a] - 13.7	109[a] - 137
	12 - 18y	147	9.5[a] - 14.8	95[a] - 148	174	9.5[a] - 13.3	95[a] - 133
3.	1 - 14d	48	12.2 - 19.9	122 - 199	35	13.6 - 18.8	136 - 188
	15 - 30d	41	9.1 - 16.9	91 - 169	34	10.5 - 15.6	105 - 156
	31 - 60d	172	8.7 - 12.7	87 - 127	130	9.4 - 13.5	94 - 135
	61 - 180d	524	9.7 - 13.3	97 - 133	388	9.9 - 13.1	99 - 131
	0.5 - <2y	2037	10.3 - 13.1	103 - 131	1691	10.4 - 13.2	104 - 132
	2 - <6y	2384	10.7 - 13.8	107 - 138	2021	10.6 - 13.8	106 - 138
	6 - <12y	1909	10.8 - 14.4	108 - 144	1785	10.6 - 14.4	106 - 144
	12 - <18y	1740	10.7 - 16.0	107 - 160	2405	10.9 - 14.6	109 - 146
	>18y	1037	9.9 – 16.5	99 - 165	2477	10.6 - 14.5	106 - 145

Specimen Type:	1,2. Whole blood (K_3/EDTA anticoagulant)
	3. Whole blood (K_2/EDTA anticoagulant)
Reference:	1, 2 Pediatric Reference Ranges, Eds. Soldin SJ, Brugnara C, et. al. 2nd Edition 1997 AACC Press.
	3. Brugnara C. Manuscript in preparation.
Method(s):	1. Bayer H*3 (Bayer Diagnostics, Tarrytown, NY)
	2. Coulter STKS (Beckman Coulter Inc., Brea, CA)
	3. Bayer ADVIA 120 (Bayer Diagnostics, Tarrytown, NY)
Comments:	1,3. Data from outpatients. A computerized approach adapted from the Hoffmann technique was utilized to remove outliers and obtain the 2.5th and 97.5th percentiles (1). The upper 90% of the data was used for the Hoffman Plot for data set 3.
	2. Data from hospitalized patients (excluding hematology, oncology, and intensive care unit patients). A computerized approach adapted from the Hoffmann technique was utilized to remove outliers and obtain the 2.5th and 97.5th percentiles.
	[a]To obtain the 2.5th percentile, the statistical technique was modified to use the central 60% of the data for the Hoffmann plot.

CELLULAR HEMOGLOBIN CONCENTRATION
DISTRIBUTION WIDTH (HDW)

Test	Age	Male		Female	
		n	g/dL	n	g/dL
1.	1 - 14d	48	2.6 - 3.5	35	2.6 - 3.2
	15 - 30d	41	2.7 - 3.3	34	2.5 - 3.0
	31 - 60d	171	2.6 - 3.7	130	2.5 - 3.5
	61 - 180d	524	2.4 - 3.3	387	2.3 - 3.2
	0.5 - <2y	2039	2.4 - 3.3	1688	2.3 - 3.2
	2 - <6y	2382	2.4 - 3.2	2020	2.3 - 3.2
	6 - <12y	1915	2.4 - 3.4	1786	2.3 - 3.3
	12 - <18y	1738	2.3 - 3.3	2402	2.2 - 3.2
	>18y	1037	2.3 - 3.6	2477	2.2 - 3.2

Specimen Type:	1. Whole blood (K_2/EDTA anticoagulant)
Reference:	1. Brugnara C. Manuscript in preparation.
Method(s):	1. Bayer ADVIA 120 (Bayer Diagnostics, Tarrytown, NY)
Comments:	1. Data from outpatients. A computerized approach adapted from the Hoffmann technique was utilized to remove outliers and obtain the 2.5th and 97.5th percentiles.

LYMPHOCYTE COUNT (ABSOLUTE)

Test	Age	Male n	Male $\times 10^3/\mu L$	Male $\times 10^9/L$	Female n	Female $\times 10^3/\mu L$	Female $\times 10^9/L$
1.	1 - 3d	47	2.2 - 5.4	2.2 - 5.4	50	2.8 - 5.3	2.8 - 5.3
	4 - 7d	32	4.3 - 7.7	4.3 - 7.7	29	4.9 - 7.0	4.9 - 7.0
	8 - 14d	39	4.2 - 7.4	4.2 - 7.4	58	4.4 - 8.3	4.4 - 8.3
	15 - 30d	137	3.9 - 8.5	3.9 - 8.5	98	4.1 - 8.9	4.1 - 8.9
	31 - 60d	463	3.3 - 8.3	3.3 - 8.3	358	3.2 - 9.1	3.2 - 9.1
	61 - 180d	1475	2.8 - 8.3	2.8 - 8.3	1166	2.8 - 8.4	2.8 - 8.4
	0.5 - <2y	5941	1.9 - 6.8	1.9 - 6.8	4608	1.2 - 7.0	1.2 - 7.0
	2 - <6y	6570	1.3 - 4.7	1.3 - 4.7	5672	1.4 - 4.7	1.4 - 4.7
	6 - <12y	5343	1.1 - 3.4	1.1 - 3.4	4719	1.1 - 3.5	1.1 - 3.5
	12 - <18y	3953	1.0 - 2.8	1.0 - 2.8	5109	1.1 - 2.8	1.1 - 2.8
	> 18y	1969	0.9 - 2.5	0.9 - 2.5	3054	1.1 - 2.7	1.1 - 2.7
2.	1 - 3d	173	0.9 - 5.5	0.9 - 5.5	114	1.2 - 5.1	1.2 - 5.1
	4 - 7d	152	1.1 - 7.8	1.1 - 7.8	108	1.3 - 5.4	1.3 - 5.4
	8 - 14d	180	1.3 - 7.5	1.3 - 7.5	124	0.8 - 8.5	0.8 - 8.5
	15 - 30d	390	0.8 - 8.3	0.8 - 8.3	291	0.9 - 8.0	0.9 - 8.0
	31 - 60d	74	1.7 - 8.4	1.7 - 8.4	184	1.2 - 8.0	1.2 - 8.0
	61 - 180d	75	1.3 - 8.8	1.3 - 8.8	102	2.1 - 7.4	2.1 - 7.4
	0.5 - <2y	177	1.1 - 6.5	1.1 - 6.5	119	1.6 - 7.5	1.6 - 7.5
	2 - <6y	189	0.5 - 4.4	0.5 - 4.4	134	1.2 - 5.0	1.2 - 5.0
	6 - <12y	126	0.8 - 3.0	0.8 - 3.0	136	0.9 - 3.4	0.9 - 3.4
	12 - 18y	140	0.4 - 2.5	0.4 - 2.5	154	0.8 - 3.2	0.8 - 3.2
3.	1 - 14d	38	3.9 - 7.2	3.9 - 7.2	28	3.0 - 6.5	3.0 - 6.5
	15 - 30d	33	3.1 - 7.0	3.1 - 7.0	27	3.2 - 7.8	3.2 - 7.8
	31 - 60d	148	2.6 - 6.8	2.6 - 6.8	109	2.2 - 7.1	2.2 - 7.1
	61 - 180d	469	2.5 - 7.8	2.5 - 7.8	357	2.3 - 7.7	2.3 - 7.7
	0.5 - <2y	1557	1.7 - 6.5	1.7 - 6.5	1257	1.7 - 6.7	1.7 - 6.7
	2 - <6y	1637	1.3 - 4.6	1.3 - 4.6	1315	1.2 - 4.5	1.2 - 4.5
	6 - <12y	1490	1.0 - 3.4	1.0 - 3.4	1391	1.2 - 3.4	1.2 - 3.4
	12 - <18y	1411	1.0 - 2.8	1.0 - 2.8	1774	1.1 - 2.8	1.1 - 2.8
	>18y	713	0.8 - 2.5	0.8 - 2.5	1077	0.9 - 2.6	0.9 - 2.6

Specimen Type:	1,2.	Whole blood (K_3/EDTA anticoagulant)
	3.	Whole blood (K_2/EDTA anticoagulant)
Reference:	1, 2	Pediatric Reference Ranges, Eds. Soldin SJ, Brugnara C, et. al. 2nd Edition 1997 AACC Press.
	3.	Brugnara C. Manuscript in preparation.
Method(s):	1.	Bayer H*3 (Bayer Diagnostics, Tarrytown, NY)
	2.	Coulter STKS (Beckman Coulter Inc., Brea, CA)
	3.	Bayer ADVIA 120 (Bayer Diagnostics, Tarrytown, NY)
Comments:	1,3.	Data from outpatients. A computerized approach adapted from the Hoffmann technique was utilized to remove outliers and obtain the 2.5th and 97.5th percentiles.
	2.	Data from hospitalized patients (excluding hematology, oncology, and intensive care unit patients). A computerized approach adapted from the Hoffmann technique was utilized to remove outliers and obtain the 2.5th and 97.5th percentiles.

LYMPHOCYTE COUNT (RELATIVE)

Test	Age	Male n	Male %	Male Number Fraction	Female n	Female %	Female Number Fraction
1.	1 - 3d	48	25.9 - 56.5	.259 - .565	50	28.4 - 54.6	.284 - .546
	4 - 7d	33	39.3 - 60.7	.393 - .607	29	38.8 - 64.1	.388 - .641
	8 - 14d	43	40.2 - 62.2	.402 - .622	58	44.6 - 67.3	.446 - .673
	15 - 30d	137	41.3 - 65.4	.413 - .654	98	35.1 - 67.4	.351 - .674
	31 - 60d	463	39.5 - 69.7	.395 - .697	359	36.7 - 69.8	.367 - .698
	61 - 180d	1475	32.0 - 68.5	.320 - .685	1165	30.4 - 68.9	.304 - .689
	0.5 - <2y	5945	19.8 - 63.7	.198 - .637	4614	19.8 - 62.8	.198 - .628
	2 - <6y	6581	14.1 - 55.0	.141 - .550	5680	15.6 - 55.6	.156 - .556
	6 - <12y	5355	14.3 - 47.9	.143 - .479	4730	13.1 - 48.4	.131 - .484
	12 - <18y	3962	13.4 - 42.8	.134 - .428	5123	14.1 - 41.3	.141 - .413
	> 18y	1970	12.8 - 43.9	.128 - .439	3062	15.4 - 39.5	.154 - .395
2.	1 - 3d	173	16.8 - 46.4	.168 - .464	114	13.4 - 40.7	.134 - .407
	4 - 7d	152	18.8 - 51.4	.188 - .514	108	18.4 - 52.9	.184 - .529
	8 - 14d	180	13.0 - 43.6	.130 - .436	124	19.0 - 54.7	.190 - .547
	15 - 30d	390	10.4 - 51.9	.104 - .519	292	17.0 - 58.7	.170 - .587
	31 - 60d	302	22.7 - 53.9	.227 - .539	184	21.3 - 63.6	.213 - .636
	61 - 180d	25	19.9 - 53.8	.199 - .538	41	25.7 - 52.9	.257 - .529
	0.5 - <2y	91	18.6 - 58.1	.186 - .581	64	16.4 - 56.3	.164 - .563
	2 - <6y	189	11.0 - 50.1	.110 - .501	134	14.3 - 50.6	.143 - .506
	6 - <12y	126	14.1 - 43.1	.141 - .431	136	13.1 - 45.2	.131 - .452
	12 - 18y	140	6.5 - 32.9	.065 - .329	154	12.9 - 40.6	.129 - .406
3.	1 - 14d	38	26.2 - 52.8	.262 - .528	28	25.0 - 51.9	.250 - .519
	15 - 30d	33	39.8 - 60.6	.398 - .606	27	34.8 - 66.5	.348 - .665
	31 - 60d	148	34.0 - 67.3	.340 - .673	109	30.4 - 64.7	.304 - .647
	61 - 180d	469	28.0 - 64.6	.280 - .646	357	24.0 - 64.0	.240 - .640
	0.5 - <2y	1557	17.0 - 61.1	.170 - .611	1258	18.4 - 61.0	.184 - .610
	2 - <6y	1637	13.5 - 52.8	.135 - .528	1317	12.5 - 51.4	.125 - .514
	6 - <12y	1491	12.2 - 44.9	.122 - .449	1395	13.7 - 43.6	.137 - .436
	12 - <18y	1415	13.0 - 41.1	.130 - .411	1770	14.5 - 39.6	.145 - .396
	>18y	713	11.5 - 36.3	.115 - .363	1079	12.1 - 35.8	.121 - .358

Specimen Type:	1,2. Whole blood (K$_3$/EDTA anticoagulant)
	3. Whole blood (K$_2$/EDTA anticoagulant)
Reference:	1, 2 Pediatric Reference Ranges, Eds. Soldin SJ, Brugnara C, et. al. 2nd Edition 1997 AACC Press.
	3. Brugnara C. Manuscript in preparation.
Method(s):	1. Bayer H*3 (Bayer Diagnostics, Tarrytown, NY)
	2. Coulter STKS (Beckman Coulter Inc., Brea, CA)
	3. Bayer ADVIA 120 (Bayer Diagnostics, Tarrytown, NY)
Comments:	1,3. Data from outpatients. A computerized approach adapted from the Hoffmann technique was utilized to remove outliers and obtain the 2.5th and 97.5th percentiles.
	2. Data from hospitalized patients (excluding hematology, oncology, and intensive care unit patients). A computerized approach adapted from the Hoffmann technique was utilized to remove outliers and obtain the 2.5th and 97.5th percentiles. To obtain the 2.5th and 97.5th percentiles, the statistical technique was modified to use the central 60% of the data for the Hoffmann plot.

MEAN CORPUSCULAR HEMOGLOBIN (MCH)

Test	Age	Male		Female	
		n	pg	n	pg
1.	1 - 3d	75	32.5 - 36.5	70	32.6 - 37.8
	4 - 7d	49	31.1 - 36.5	38	32.2 - 36.6
	8 - 14d	61	30.6 - 35.7	69	31.7 - 36.5
	15 - 30d	168	30.1 - 33.8	116	30.8 - 34.6
	31 - 60d	561	28.4 - 32.6	420	28.6 - 32.9
	61 - 180d	1838	24.5 - 29.1	1362	24.7 - 29.6
	0.5 - <2y	8842	23.2 - 27.5	6926	23.5 - 27.6
	2 - <6y	11140	24.1 - 28.4	9746	24.3 - 28.6
	6 - <12y	7465	25.4 - 29.4	6806	25.4 - 29.6
	12 - <18y	5545	25.8 - 30.3	7993	26.1 - 30.4
	> 18y	3171	27.2 - 31.7	8604	26.2 - 31.0
2.	1 - 3d	174	31.3 - 38.6	115	31.4 - 39.4
	4 - 7d	155	29.9 - 36.2	108	30.8 - 36.8
	8 - 14d	182	29.1 - 35.7	124	30.3 - 35.0
	15 - 30d	393	28.8 - 33.6	291	29.2 - 34.3
	31 - 60d	74	28.0 - 30.5	185	29.0 - 32.7
	61 - 180d	75	25.8 - 29.2	102	25.8 - 30.1
	0.5 - <2y	177	24.2 - 30.0	119	23.4 - 30.0
	2 - <6y	190	24.6 - 30.9	135	25.3 - 29.9
	6 - <12y	128	26.3 - 30.3	138	27.4 - 33.2
	12 - 18y	140	25.9 - 31.0	154	26.7 - 31.7
3.	1 - 14d	48	32.2 - 35.4	35	32.4 - 36.5
	15 - 30d	41	30.0 - 33.7	34	29.7 - 34.4
	31 - 60d	172	28.6 - 31.8	130	28.6 - 32.2
	61 - 180d	524	24.2 - 29.0	386	24.8 - 29.2
	0.5 - <2y	2039	23.2 - 27.3	1686	23.4 - 27.4
	2 - <6y	2382	24.2 - 28.1	2019	24.1 - 28.5
	6 - <12y	1912	25.6 - 29.4	1788	25.2 - 29.7
	12 - <18y	1740	25.7 - 30.2	2403	25.9 - 30.2
	>18y	1038	27.1 - 31.8	2479	25.8 - 31.3

Specimen Type:	1,2. Whole blood (K_3/EDTA anticoagulant)
	3. Whole blood (K_2/EDTA anticoagulant)
Reference:	1, 2 Pediatric Reference Ranges, Eds. Soldin SJ, Brugnara C, et. al. 2nd Edition 1997 AACC Press.
	3. Brugnara C. Manuscript in preparation.
Method(s):	1. Bayer H*3 (Bayer Diagnostics, Tarrytown, NY)
	2. Coulter STKS (Beckman Coulter Inc., Brea, CA)
	3. Bayer ADVIA 120 (Bayer Diagnostics, Tarrytown, NY)
Comments:	1,3. Data from outpatients. A computerized approach adapted from the Hoffmann technique was utilized to remove outliers and obtain the 2.5th and 97.5th percentiles.
	2. Data from hospitalized patients (excluding hematology, oncology, and intensive care unit patients). A computerized approach adapted from the Hoffmann technique was utilized to remove outliers and obtain the 2.5th and 97.5th percentiles.

MEAN CORPUSCULAR HEMOGLOBIN CONCENTRATION (MCHC)

Test	Age	Male			Female		
		n	%	Concentration Fraction	n	%	Concentration Fraction
1.	1 - 3d	76	32.1 - 34.2	.321 - .342	76	31.6 - 34.7	.316 - .347
	4 - 7d	49	32.0 - 34.6	.320 - .346	39	31.8 - 34.6	.318 - .346
	8 - 14d	60	32.0 - 35.0	.320 - .350	69	32.1 - 34.8	.321 - .348
	15 - 30d	167	32.3 - 35.0	.323 - .350	116	32.0 - 35.0	.320 - .350
	31 - 60d	562	32.5 - 35.5	.325 - .355	419	32.2 - 35.3	.322 - .353
	61 - 180d	1389	32.0 - 35.1	.320 - .351	1363	32.0 - 35.1	.320 - .351
	0.5 - <2y	8856	31.9 - 35.0	.319 - .350	6931	31.8 - 34.8	.318 - .348
	2 - <6y	11149	31.9 - 35.1	.319 - .351	9744	31.9 - 35.0	.319 - .350
	6 - <12y	7465	32.2 - 35.2	.322 - .352	6803	31.9 - 35.0	.319 - .350
	12 - <18y	5545	31.8 - 35.0	.318 - .350	7991	31.6 - 34.7	.316 - .347
	> 18y	3170	31.9 - 35.1	.319 - .351	8607	31.4 - 34.3	.314 - .343
2.	1 - 3d	174	33.5 - 34.8	.335 - .348	115	33.3 - 34.5	.333 - .345
	4 - 7d	155	33.5 - 35.0	.335 - .350	108	33.6 - 35.0	.336 - .350
	8 - 14d	182	33.5 - 35.0	.335 - .350	124	33.5 - 35.2	.335 - .352
	15 - 30d	393	33.5 - 35.0	.335 - .350	291	33.5 - 35.0	.335 - .350
	31 - 60d	74	33.5 - 34.6	.335 - .346	185	33.5 - 34.8	.335 - .348
	61 - 180d	75	32.9 - 34.0	.329 - .340	102	33.1 - 34.4	.331 - .344
	0.5 - <2y	177	32.9 - 34.5	.329 - .345	119	32.7 - 34.6	.327 - .346
	2 - <6y	190	32.7 - 34.7	.327 - .347	135	32.9 - 34.6	.329 - .346
	6 - <12y	128	33.2 - 34.8	.332 - .348	138	33.3 - 34.8	.333 - .348
	12 - 18y	140	33.4 - 34.6	.334 - .346	154	33.2 - 34.7	.332 - .347
3.	1 - 14d	48	32.8 - 35.3	.328 - .353	35	32.9 - 34.4	.329 - .344
	15 - 30d	41	33.0 - 35.3	.330 - .353	34	33.3 - 35.1	.333 - .351
	31 - 60d	172	33.0 - 35.8	.330 - .358	130	33.4 - 35.5	.334 - .355
	61 - 180d	524	32.6 - 35.3	.326 - .353	388	32.6 - 35.4	.326 - .354
	0.5 - <2y	2041	32.4 - 35.0	.324 - .350	1690	32.4 - 34.9	.324 - .349
	2 - <6y	2386	32.8 - 35.3	.328 - .353	2022	32.4 - 35.1	.324 - .351
	6 - <12y	1917	32.8 - 35.3	.328 - .353	1789	32.3 - 35.2	.323 - .352
	12 - <18y	1740	32.3 - 35.2	.323 - .352	2405	32.0 - 34.7	.320 - .347
	>18y	1038	32.0 - 34.9	.320 - .349	2478	31.6 - 34.4	.316 - .344

Specimen Type:	1,2. Whole blood (K_3/EDTA anticoagulant)
	3. Whole blood (K_2/EDTA anticoagulant)
Reference:	1, 2 Pediatric Reference Ranges, Eds. Soldin SJ, Brugnara C, et. al. 2nd Edition 1997 AACC Press.
	3. Brugnara C. Manuscript in preparation.
Method(s):	1. Bayer H*3 (Bayer Diagnostics, Tarrytown, NY)
	2. Coulter STKS (Beckman Coulter Inc., Brea, CA)
	3. Bayer ADVIA 120 (Bayer Diagnostics, Tarrytown, NY)
Comments:	1,3. Data from outpatients. A computerized approach adapted from the Hoffmann technique was utilized to remove outliers and obtain the 2.5th and 97.5th percentiles.
	2. Data from hospitalized patients (excluding hematology, oncology, and intensive care unit patients). A computerized approach adapted from the Hoffmann technique was utilized to remove outliers and obtain the 2.5th and 97.5th percentiles.

MEAN CORPUSCULAR VOLUME (MCV)

Test	Age	Male n	Male μm³	Male fL	Female n	Female μm³	Female fL
1.	1 - 3d	76	97.3 - 109.8	97.3 - 109.8	76	99.4 - 113.8	99.4 - 113.8
	4 - 7d	49	95.5 - 109.3	95.5 - 109.3	39	97.9 - 111.6	97.9 - 111.6
	8 - 14d	61	93.1 - 105.4	93.1 - 105.4	69	97.3 - 109.3	97.3 - 109.3
	15 - 30d	168	88.7 - 101.2	88.7 - 101.2	116	91.8 - 102.5	91.8 - 102.5
	31 - 60d	562	84.6 - 95.4	84.6 - 95.4	418	85.0 - 96.9	85.0 - 96.9
	61 - 180d	1841	73.6 - 86.6	73.6 - 86.6	1363	74.7 - 87.6	74.7 - 87.6
	0.5 - <2y	8852	70.5 - 81.2	70.5 - 81.2	6927	71.5 - 81.8	71.5 - 81.8
	2 - <6y	11149	72.7 - 83.6	72.7 - 83.6	9750	73.8 - 84.3	73.8 - 84.3
	6 - <12y	7467	75.9 - 86.5	75.9 - 86.5	6795	76.8 - 87.6	76.8 - 87.6
	12 - <18y	5551	77.9 - 89.8	77.9 - 89.8	7995	79.4 - 91.0	79.4 - 91.0
	> 18y	3173	81.3 - 94.2	81.3 - 94.2	8608	80.8 - 93.4	80.8 - 93.4
2.	1 - 3d	174	93.0 - 113.4	93.0 - 113.4	117	92.4 - 115.4	92.4 - 115.4
	4 - 7d	155	88.1 - 106.5	88.1 - 106.5	108	90.6 - 108.3	90.6 - 108.3
	8 - 14d	182	85.1 - 104.5	85.1 - 104.5	124	87.9 - 101.8	87.9 - 101.8
	15 - 30d	393	83.4 - 97.6	83.4 - 97.6	291	84.5 - 99.7	84.5 - 99.7
	31 - 60d	74	82.0 - 89.8	82.0 - 89.8	185	85.5 - 95.3	85.5 - 95.3
	61 - 180d	75	76.5 - 87.8	76.5 - 87.8	102	77.5 - 89.4	77.5 - 89.4
	0.5 - <2y	177	72.3 - 88.7	72.3 - 88.7	119	70.6 - 87.9	70.6 - 87.9
	2 - <6y	190	73.6 - 90.0	73.6 - 90.0	135	75.6 - 88.0	75.6 - 88.0
	6 - <12y	128	77.3 - 88.3	77.3 - 88.3	138	80.7 - 95.6	80.7 - 95.6
	12 - 18y	140	76.3 - 90.1	76.3 - 90.1	154	79.1 - 91.7	79.1 - 91.7
3.	1 - 14d	48	95.9 - 100.9	95.9 - 100.9	35	98.0 - 104.2	98.0 - 104.2
	15 - 30d	41	80.3 - 100.1	80.3 - 100.1	34	88.9 - 98.4	88.9 - 98.4
	31 - 60d	172	83.9 - 91.8	83.9 - 91.8	130	82.9 - 93.8	82.9 - 93.8
	61 - 180d	524	71.8 - 85.1	71.8 - 85.1	389	73.8 - 85.8	73.8 - 85.8
	0.5 - <2y	2041	69.5 - 79.7	69.5 - 79.7	1689	70.9 - 80.1	70.9 - 80.1
	2 - <6y	2385	72.4 - 82.2	72.4 - 82.2	2022	72.7 - 83.1	72.7 - 83.1
	6 - <12y	1917	75.1 - 85.9	75.1 - 85.9	1784	75.6 - 86.8	75.6 - 86.8
	12 - <18y	1740	76.9 - 88.8	76.9 - 88.8	2402	78.3 - 89.7	78.3 - 89.7
	>18y	1038	80.6 - 95.0	80.6 - 95.0	2478	79.5 - 93.9	79.5 - 93.9

211

Specimen Type:	1,2. Whole blood (K_3/EDTA anticoagulant) 3. Whole blood (K_2/EDTA anticoagulant)
Reference:	1, 2 Pediatric Reference Ranges, Eds. Soldin SJ, Brugnara C, et. al. 2nd Edition 1997 AACC Press. 3. Brugnara C. Manuscript in preparation.
Method(s):	1. Bayer H*3 (Bayer Diagnostics, Tarrytown, NY) 2. Coulter STKS (Beckman Coulter Inc., Brea, CA) 3. Bayer ADVIA 120 (Bayer Diagnostics, Tarrytown, NY)
Comments:	1,3. Data from outpatients. A computerized approach adapted from the Hoffmann technique was utilized to remove outliers and obtain the 2.5th and 97.5th percentiles. 2. Data from hospitalized patients (excluding hematology, oncology, and intensive care unit patients). A computerized approach adapted from the Hoffmann technique was utilized to remove outliers and obtain the 2.5th and 97.5th percentiles.

MEAN PLATELET VOLUME (MPV)

Test	Age	Male			Female		
		n	μm^3	fL	n	μm^3	fL
1.	1 - 3d	170	7.1 - 8.4	7.1 - 8.4	115	7.3 - 8.6	7.3 - 8.6
	4 - 7d	151	7.5 - 9.2	7.5 - 9.2	107	7.8 - 9.3	7.8 - 9.3
	8 - 14d	179	8.1 - 10.0	8.1 - 10.0	124	8.2 - 10.1	8.2 - 10.1
	15 - 30d	387	8.0 - 10.6	8.0 - 10.6	287	8.0 - 10.9	8.0 - 10.9
	31 - 60d	74	7.0 - 11.3	7.0 - 11.3	184	7.4 - 9.7	7.4 - 9.7
	61 - 180d	75	6.8 - 9.0	6.8 - 9.0	102	7.2 - 8.9	7.2 - 8.9
	0.5 - <2y	177	7.1 - 9.3	7.1 - 9.3	119	7.0 - 9.3	7.0 - 9.3
	2 - <6y	190	7.1 - 9.3	7.1 - 9.3	135	6.9 - 8.8	6.9 - 8.8
	6 - <12y	127	7.2 - 9.4	7.2 - 9.4	135	7.1 - 9.2	7.1 - 9.2
	12 - <18y	140	7.3 - 9.7	7.3 - 9.7	154	7.5 - 9.3	7.5 - 9.3
2.	1 - 14d	46	7.6 - 9.9	7.6 - 9.9	35	7.5 - 9.3	7.5 - 9.3
	15 - 30d	47	7.1 - 9.9	7.1 - 9.9	36	7.7 - 9.4	7.7 - 9.4
	31 - 60d	167	7.4 - 9.1	7.4 - 9.1	129	7.5 - 9.5	7.5 - 9.5
	61 - 180d	534	7.2 - 9.0	7.2 - 9.0	390	7.2 - 8.8	7.2 - 8.8
	0.5 - <2y	2056	7.0 - 8.8	7.0 - 8.8	1709	7.1 - 8.8	7.1 - 8.8
	2 - <6y	2423	7.1 - 8.9	7.1 - 8.9	2059	7.1 - 8.9	7.1 - 8.9
	6 - <12y	1933	7.3 - 9.1	7.3 - 9.1	1833	7.3 - 9.3	7.3 - 9.3
	12 - <18y	1802	7.5 - 9.6	7.5 - 9.6	2458	7.5 - 9.6	7.5 - 9.6
	>18y	1039	7.6 - 9.6	7.6 - 9.6	2526	7.7 - 9.8	7.7 - 9.8

Specimen Type:	1. Whole blood (K_3/EDTA anticoagulant)
	2. Whole blood (K_2/EDTA anticoagulant)
Reference:	1. Pediatric Reference Ranges, Eds. Soldin SJ, Brugnara C, et. al. 2nd Edition 1997 AACC Press.
	2. Brugnara C. Manuscript in preparation.
Method(s):	1. Coulter STKS (Beckman Coulter Inc., Brea, CA)
	2. Bayer ADVIA 120 (Bayer Diagnostics, Tarrytown, NY)
Comments:	1. Data from hospitalized patients (excluding hematology, oncology, and intensive care unit patients). A computerized approach adapted from the Hoffmann technique was utilized to remove outliers and obtain the 2.5th and 97.5th percentiles.
	2. Data from outpatients. A computerized approach adapted from the Hoffmann technique was utilized to remove outliers and obtain the 2.5th and 97.5th percentiles.

MONOCYTE COUNT (ABSOLUTE)

Test	Age	Male n	Male × 10³/μL	Male × 10⁹/L	Female n	Female × 10³/μL	Female × 10⁹/L
1.	1 - 3d	172	0.2 - 1.8	0.2 - 1.8	114	0.2 - 2.2	0.2 - 2.2
	4 - 7d	152	0.2 - 2.2	0.2 - 2.2	108	0.2 - 2.2	0.2 - 2.2
	8 - 14d	180	0.3 - 3.0	0.3 - 3.0	124	0.1 - 2.9	0.1 - 2.9
	15 - 30d	390	0.2 - 3.5	0.2 - 3.5	290	0.2 - 5.0	0.2 - 5.0
	31 - 60d	74	0.3 - 2.7	0.3 - 2.7	184	0.2 - 2.1	0.2 - 2.1
	61 - 180d	75	0.5 - 1.9	0.5 - 1.9	102	0.6 - 1.9	0.6 - 1.9
	0.5 - <2y	177	0.4 - 2.0	0.4 - 2.0	119	0.3 - 1.5	0.3 - 1.5
	2 - <6y	189	0.3 - 1.2	0.3 - 1.2	134	0.5 - 1.1	0.5 - 1.1
	6 - <12y	126	0.3 - 0.9	0.3 - 0.9	136	0.4 - 0.9	0.4 - 0.9
	12 - 18y	140	0.4 - 1.3	0.4 - 1.3	154	0.4 - 0.9	0.4 - 0.9

Specimen Type:	Whole blood (K$_3$/EDTA anticoagulant)
Reference:	Pediatric Reference Ranges, Eds. Soldin SJ, Brugnara C, et. al. 2nd Edition 1997 AACC Press.
Method(s):	Coulter STKS (Beckman Coulter Inc., Brea, CA)
Comments:	Data from hospitalized patients (excluding hematology, oncology, and intensive care unit patients). A computerized approach adapted from the Hoffmann technique was utilized to remove outliers and obtain the 2.5th and 97.5th percentiles.

MONOCYTE COUNT (RELATIVE)

Test	Age	Male			Female		
		n	%	Number Fraction	n	%	Number Fraction
1.	1 - 3d	48	6.8 - 13.3	.068 - .133	50	7.6 - 13.2	.076 - .132
	4 - 7d	33	8.2 - 13.1	.082 - .131	29	5.9 - 12.0	.059 - .120
	8 - 14d	43	6.3 - 13.4	.063 - .134	58	6.9 - 13.5	.069 - .135
	15 - 30d	137	7.1 - 13.7	.071 - .137	98	6.0 - 15.9	.060 - .159
	31 - 60d	463	6.3 - 13.7	.063 - .137	359	5.6 - 13.9	.056 - .139
	61 - 180d	1475	5.0 - 12.6	.050 - .126	1166	4.8 - 12.4	.048 - .124
	0.5 - <2y	5944	4.6 - 11.2	.046 - .112	4614	4.4 - 10.6	.044 - .106
	2 - <6y	6580	4.3 - 8.9	.043 - .089	3419	4.1 - 8.7	.041 - .087
	6 - <12y	5356	4.4 - 8.7	.044 - .087	4729	4.0 - 8.0	.040 - .080
	12 - <18y	3959	4.7 - 9.1	.047 - .091	5121	4.1 - 8.0	.041 - .080
	> 18y	1970	4.8 - 9.4	.048 - .094	3060	4.2 - 7.9	.042 - .079
2.	1 - 3d	172	0.8 - 11.9	.008 - .119	114	1.4 - 16.3	.014 - .163
	4 - 7d	152	1.7 - 18.7	.017 - .187	108	1.3 - 18.7	.013 - .187
	8 - 14d	180	1.9 - 20.8	.019 - .208	124	2.3 - 22.2	.023 - .222
	15 - 30d	390	1.0 - 20.9	.010 - .209	290	2.7 - 22.9	.027 - .229
	31 - 60d	74	4.9 - 19.6	.049 - .196	184	2.4 - 19.1	.024 - .191
	61 - 180d	75	2.3 - 17.3	.023 - .173	102	4.6 - 18.1	.046 - .181
	0.5 - <2y	177	4.6 - 15.4	.046 - .154	119	3.3 - 15.5	.033 - .155
	2 - <6y	189	3.5 - 13.9	.035 - .139	134	5.7 - 13.2	.057 - .132
	6 - <12y	126	3.3 - 13.4	.033 - .134	136	4.2 - 12.3	.042 - .123
	12 - 18y	140	3.1 - 12.5	.031 - .125	154	3.8 - 11.2	.038 - .112
3.	1 - 14d	38	9.1 - 13.9	.091 - .139	28	7.1 - 12.0	.071 - .120
	15 - 30d	33	7.7 - 13.8	.077 - .138	27	5.5 - 13.3	.055 - .133
	31 - 60d	147	5.9 - 13.9	.059 - .139	109	6.0 - 12.0	.060 - .120
	61 - 180d	469	4.5 - 11.4	.045 - .114	357	4.4 - 11.1	.044 - .111
	0.5 - <2y	1558	4.1 - 10.2	.041 - .102	1258	3.6 - 9.0	.036 - .090
	2 - <6y	1637	3.5 - 7.8	.035 - .078	1317	3.3 - 7.5	.033 - .075
	6 - <12y	1491	3.7 - 7.9	.037 - .079	1395	3.3 - 7.4	.033 - .074
	12 - <18y	1415	3.8 - 8.2	.038 - .082	1771	3.5 - 7.2	.035 - .072
	>18y	713	4.1 - 8.6	.041 - .086	1077	3.4 - 7.0	.034 - .070

Specimen Type:	1,2. Whole blood (K_3/EDTA anticoagulant)
	3. Whole blood (K_2/EDTA anticoagulant)
Reference:	1, 2 Pediatric Reference Ranges, Eds. Soldin SJ, Brugnara C, et. al. 2nd Edition 1997 AACC Press.
	3. Brugnara C. Manuscript in preparation.
Method(s):	1. Bayer H*3 (Bayer Diagnostics, Tarrytown, NY)
	2. Coulter STKS (Beckman Coulter Inc., Brea, CA)
	3. Bayer ADVIA 120 (Bayer Diagnostics, Tarrytown, NY)
Comments:	1,3. Data from outpatients. A computerized approach adapted from the Hoffmann technique was utilized to remove outliers and obtain the 2.5th and 97.5th percentiles.
	2. Data from hospitalized patients (excluding hematology, oncology, and intensive care unit patients). A computerized approach adapted from the Hoffmann technique was utilized to remove outliers and obtain the 2.5th and 97.5th percentiles.

NEUTROPHIL COUNT (ABSOLUTE)

Test	Age	n	× 10³/μL	× 10⁹/L	n	× 10³/μL	× 10⁹/L
			Male			Female	
1.	1 - 3d	48	1.7 - 4.7	1.7 - 4.7	50	2.1 - 8.4	2.1 - 8.4
	4 - 7d	32	1.9 - 4.1	1.9 - 4.1	29	1.8 - 5.1	1.8 - 5.1
	8 - 14d	43	1.9 - 5.2	1.9 - 5.2	58	1.7 - 5.4	1.7 - 5.4
	15 - 30d	137	1.5 - 3.6	1.5 - 3.6	98	1.3 - 4.3	1.3 - 4.3
	31 - 60d	463	1.2 - 4.4	1.2 - 4.4	359	1.2 - 4.9	1.2 - 4.9
	61 - 180d	1475	1.4 - 6.4	1.4 - 6.4	1166	1.4 - 6.7	1.4 - 6.7
	0.5 - <2y	5941	1.6 - 8.3	1.6 - 8.3	4607	1.8 - 9.1	1.8 - 9.1
	2 - <6y	6571	1.8 - 7.4	1.8 - 7.4	5674	1.8 - 6.8	1.8 - 6.8
	6 - <12y	5346	1.8 - 6.6	1.8 - 6.6	4721	1.8 - 6.7	1.8 - 6.7
	12 - <18y	3954	2.0 - 6.6	2.0 - 6.6	5110	2.3 - 6.9	2.3 - 6.9
	> 18y	1969	2.1 - 6.5	2.1 - 6.5	3055	2.5 - 7.0	2.5 - 7.0
2.	1 - 3d	173	2.7 - 9.0	2.7 - 9.0	114	3.4 - 11.3	3.4 - 11.3
	4 - 7d	152	1.8 - 7.1	1.8 - 7.1	108	2.2 - 7.2	2.2 - 7.2
	8 - 14d	180	3.2 - 11.4	3.2 - 11.4	124	1.7 - 7.6	1.7 - 7.6
	15 - 30d	390	1.6 - 8.7	1.6 - 8.7	291	1.6 - 10.7	1.6 - 10.7
	31 - 60d	302	1.7 - 6.0	1.7 - 6.0	184	1.5 - 5.8	1.5 - 5.8
	61 - 180d	75	1.2 - 5.7	1.2 - 5.7	102	2.2 - 8.4	2.2 - 8.4
	0.5 - <2y	177	2.4 - 9.0	2.4 - 9.0	119	1.4 - 5.2	1.4 - 5.2
	2 - <6y	189	2.0 - 7.1	2.0 - 7.1	134	2.2 - 5.7	2.2 - 5.7
	6 - <12y	126	2.3 - 7.8	2.3 - 7.8	136	2.0 - 7.2	2.0 - 7.2
	12 - 18y	140	2.8 - 11.1	2.8 - 11.1	154	2.3 - 6.7	2.3 - 6.7
3.	1 - 14d	38	2.1 – 7.5	2.1 – 7.5	27	2.2 - 4.1	2.2 - 4.1
	15 - 30d	37	1.7 - 4.1	1.7 - 4.1	29	1.8 - 2.9	1.8 - 2.9
	31 - 60d	148	1.1 - 3.2	1.1 - 3.2	111	1.3 - 3.8	1.3 - 3.8
	61 - 180d	472	1.4 - 6.7	1.4 - 6.7	361	1.7 - 7.9	1.7 - 7.9
	0.5 - <2y	1569	1.8 - 9.4	1.8 - 9.4	1271	1.9 - 9.6	1.9 - 9.6
	2 - <6y	1651	2.1 - 7.9	2.1 - 7.9	1326	2.1 - 8.9	2.1 - 8.9
	6 - <12y	1503	2.1 - 7.3	2.1 - 7.3	1403	2.1 - 7.8	2.1 - 7.8
	12 - <18y	1429	2.1 - 7.0	2.1 - 7.0	1788	2.5 - 7.1	2.5 - 7.1
	>18y	716	2.3 - 7.4	2.3 - 7.6	1092	2.5 - 7.5	2.5 - 7.5

| Specimen Type: | 1,2. Whole blood (K$_3$/EDTA anticoagulant) |
	3. Whole blood (K$_2$/EDTA anticoagulant)
Reference:	1, 2 Pediatric Reference Ranges, Eds. Soldin SJ, Brugnara C, et. al. 2nd Edition 1997 AACC Press.
	3. Brugnara C. Manuscript in preparation.
Method(s):	1. Bayer H*3 (Bayer Diagnostics, Tarrytown, NY)
	2. Coulter STKS (Beckman Coulter Inc., Brea, CA)
	3. Bayer ADVIA 120 (Bayer Diagnostics, Tarrytown, NY)
Comments:	1,3. Data from outpatients. A computerized approach adapted from the Hoffmann technique was utilized to remove outliers and obtain the 2.5th and 97.5th percentiles.
	2. Data from hospitalized patients (excluding hematology, oncology, and intensive care unit patients). A computerized approach adapted from the Hoffmann technique was utilized to remove outliers and obtain the 2.5th and 97.5th percentiles. To obtain the 2.5th and 97.5th percentiles, the statistical technique was modified to use the central 60% of the data for the Hoffmann plot.

NEUTROPHIL COUNT (RELATIVE)

Test	Age	Male n	Male %	Male Number Fraction	Female n	Female %	Female Number Fraction
1.	1 - 3d	48	24.1 - 50.3	.241 - .503	50	23.1 - 58.4	.231 - .584
	4 - 7d	33	18.4 - 36.3	.184 - .363	29	18.0 - 35.0	.180 - .350
	8 - 14d	43	18.3 - 36.3	.183 - .363	58	17.1 - 33.1	.171 - .331
	15 - 30d	137	14.7 - 35.3	.147 - .353	98	13.5 - 41.6	.135 - .416
	31 - 60d	462	14.2 - 40.0	.142 - .400	359	13.6 - 44.5	.136 - .445
	61 - 180d	1475	16.3 - 51.6	.163 - .516	1166	16.3 - 53.6	.163 - .536
	0.5 - <2y	5946	21.3 - 66.7	.213 - .667	4615	22.2 - 67.1	.222 - .671
	2 - <6y	6580	30.3 - 74.3	.303 - .743	5680	30.4 - 73.3	.304 - .733
	6 - <12y	5356	36.3 - 74.3	.363 - .743	4730	37.4 - 77.1	.374 - .771
	12 - <18y	3959	41.2 - 75.5	.412 - .755	5124	45.0 - 76.4	.450 - .764
	>18y	1970	38.9 - 75.1	.389 - .751	3062	47.0 - 74.6	.470 - .746
2.	1 - 3d	172	32.2 - 69.8	.322 - .698	114	33.9 - 69.6	.339 - .696
	4 - 7d	152	25.6 - 67.7	.256 - .677	108	21.6 - 59.0	.216 - .590
	8 - 14d	180	29.0 - 65.9	.290 - .659	124	15.8 - 61.1	.158 - .611
	15 - 30d	390	18.7 - 58.8	.187 - .588	291	17.3 - 61.0	.173 - .610
	31 - 60d	302	17.1 - 51.0	.171 - .510	184	16.0 - 58.9	.160 - .589
	61 - 180d	75	11.9 - 53.4	.119 - .534	102	21.8 - 61.2	.218 - .612
	0.5 - <2y	177	24.6 - 70.9	.246 - .709	119	20.7 - 61.8	.207 - .618
	2 - <6y	189	34.3 - 78.6	.343 - .786	134	32.3 - 69.7	.323 - .697
	6 - <12y	126	40.3 - 72.9	.403 - .729	136	39.5 - 76.9	.395 - .769
	12 - 18y	140	48.5 - 85.1	.485 - .851	154	41.9 - 77.8	.419 - .778
3.	1 - 14d	38	24.1 - 47.1	.241 - .471	27	21.2 - 55.4	.212 - .554
	15 - 30d	37	18.4 - 32.4	.184 - .324	29	17.0 - 40.9	.170 - .409
	31 - 60d	148	14.6 - 40.9	.146 - .409	111	15.7 - 49.1	.157 - .491
	61 - 180d	472	17.0 - 55.5	.170 - .555	361	18.6 - 60.0	.186 - .600
	0.5 - <2y	1571	22.7 - 69.2	.227 - .692	1272	23.8 - 69.3	.238 - .693
	2 - <6y	1651	31.7 - 75.4	.317 - .754	1328	33.6 - 77.5	.336 - .775
	6 - <12y	1503	38.8 - 76.7	.388 - .767	1406	38.7 - 76.7	.387 - .767
	12 - <18y	1433	43.2 - 76.7	.432 - .767	1786	46.4 - 75.6	.464 - .756
	>18y	716	47.2 - 77.6	.472 - .776	1094	50.4 - 77.7	.504 - 777

Specimen Type:	1,2. Whole blood (K_3/EDTA anticoagulant) 3. Whole blood (K_2/EDTA anticoagulant)
Reference:	1, 2 Pediatric Reference Ranges, Eds. Soldin SJ, Brugnara C, et. al. 2nd Edition 1997 AACC Press. 3. Brugnara C. Manuscript in preparation.
Method(s):	1. Bayer H*3 (Bayer Diagnostics, Tarrytown, NY) 2. Coulter STKS (Beckman Coulter Inc., Brea, CA) 3. Bayer ADVIA 120 (Bayer Diagnostics, Tarrytown, NY)
Comments:	1,3. Data from outpatients. A computerized approach adapted from the Hoffmann technique was utilized to remove outliers and obtain the 2.5th and 97.5th percentiles. 2. Data from hospitalized patients (excluding hematology, oncology, and intensive care unit patients). A computerized approach adapted from the Hoffmann technique was utilized to remove outliers and obtain the 2.5th and 97.5th percentiles. To obtain the 2.5th and 97.5th percentiles, the statistical technique was modified to use the central 60% of the data for the Hoffmann plot.

PLASMA FIBRINOGEN

Test	Age	Male			Female		
		n	mg/dL	g/L	n	mg/dL	g/L
1.	1d - 18y	131	150 - 302	1.50 - 3.02	96	184 - 366	1.84 - 3.66
2.	1d - 18y	204	119 - 346	1.19 - 3.46	146	116 - 293	1.16 - 2.93

Specimen Type:	1, 2 Plasma (citrate anticoagulant)
Reference:	1, 2 Pediatric Reference Ranges, Eds. Soldin SJ, Brugnara C, et. al. 2nd Edition 1997 AACC Press.
Method(s):	1. Reagents: Dade® Thromboplastin C+ (Dade International, Bedford, MA) Instrumentation: Electra 1000C (Hemoliance, Pleasantville, NY) 2. Reagents: (Instrumentation Laboratories, Lexington, MA) Instrumentation: ACL 1000 (Instrumentation Laboratories, Lexington, MA)
Comments:	1. Data from outpatients. A computerized approach adapted from the Hoffmann technique was utilized to remove outliers and obtain the 2.5th and 97.5th percentiles. 2. Data from hospitalized patients (excluding hematology, oncology, and intensive care unit patients). A computerized approach adapted from the Hoffmann technique was utilized to remove outliers and obtain the 2.5th and 97.5th percentiles.

PLATELET COUNT

Test	Age	Male n	Male ×10³/μL	Male ×10⁹/L	Female n	Female ×10³/μL	Female ×10⁹/L
1.	1 - 3d	55	164 - 351	164 - 351	60	234 - 346	234 - 346
	4 - 7d	32	220 - 411	220 - 411	32	126 - 462	126 - 462
	8 - 14d	48	226 - 587	226 - 587	59	265 - 557	265 - 557
	15 - 30d	138	210 - 493	210 - 493	99	236 - 554	236 - 554
	31 - 60d	442	275 - 567	275 - 567	339	295 - 615	295 - 615
	61 - 180d	1393	275 - 566	275 - 566	1100	288 - 598	288 - 598
	0.5 - <2y	6248	219 - 452	219 - 452	4830	229 - 465	229 - 465
	2 - <6y	7576	204 - 405	204 - 405	6530	204 - 402	204 - 402
	6 - <12y	5450	194 - 364	194 - 364	4941	183 - 369	183 - 369
	12 - <18y	3935	165 - 332	165 - 332	5478	185 - 335	185 - 335
	> 18y	2048	143 - 320	143 - 320	4899	171 - 326	171 - 326
2.	1 - 3d	171	145[a] - 262	145[a] - 262	115	158[a] - 300	158[a] - 300
	4 - 7d	151	128[a] - 309	128[a] - 309	107	108[a] - 354	108[a] - 354
	8 - 14d	179	124[a] - 367	124[a] - 367	124	136[a] - 411	136[a] - 411
	15 - 30d	386	153[a] - 403	153[a] - 403	288	122[a] - 492	122[a] - 492
	31 - 60d	302	140[b] - 557	140[b] - 557	185	192[b] - 574	192[b] - 574
	61 - 180d	75	270[b] - 505[c]	270[b] - 505[c]	102	135[b] - 488[c]	135[b] - 488[c]
	0.5 - <2y	177	200[b] - 402[c]	200[b] - 402[c]	119	238[b] - 444[c]	238[b] - 444[c]
	2 - <6y	190	197[b] - 382[c]	197[b] - 382[c]	135	213[b] - 363[c]	213[b] - 363[c]
	6 - <12y	126	175[b] - 311[c]	175[b] - 311[c]	135	130[b] - 314[c]	130[b] - 314[c]
	12 - 18y	140	159 - 353	159 - 353	154	138 - 345	138 - 345
3.	1 - 14d	45	249 - 481	249 - 481	34	236 - 441	236 - 441
	15 - 30d	45	253 - 493	253 - 493	36	315 - 506	315 - 506
	31 - 60d	165	269 - 591	269 - 591	129	320 - 608	320 - 608
	61 - 180d	524	307 - 619	307 - 619	387	304 - 574	304 - 574
	0.5 - <2y	2032	229 - 494	229 - 494	1684	238 - 497	238 - 497
	2 - <6y	2382	228 - 433	228 - 433	2022	229 - 435	229 - 435
	6 - <12y	1904	209 - 405	209 - 405	1779	204 - 406	204 - 406
	12 - <18y	1751	179 - 360	179 - 360	2410	201 - 363	201 - 363
	>18y	1025	153 - 337	153 - 337	2496	177 - 354	177 - 354

Specimen Type:	1,2.	Whole blood (K_3/EDTA anticoagulant)
	3.	Whole blood (K_2/EDTA anticoagulant)
Reference:	1, 2	Pediatric Reference Ranges, Eds. Soldin SJ, Brugnara C, et. al. 2nd Edition 1997 AACC Press.
	3.	Brugnara C. Manuscript in preparation.
Method(s):	1.	Bayer H*3 (Bayer Diagnostics, Tarrytown, NY)
	2.	Coulter STKS (Beckman Coulter Inc., Brea, CA)
	3.	Bayer ADVIA 120 (Bayer Diagnostics, Tarrytown, NY)
Comments:	1,3.	Data from outpatients. A computerized approach adapted from the Hoffmann technique was utilized to remove outliers and obtain the 2.5th and 97.5th percentiles.
	2.	Data from hospitalized patients (excluding hematology, oncology, and intensive care unit patients). A computerized approach adapted from the Hoffmann technique was utilized to remove outliers and obtain the 2.5th and 97.5th percentiles. [a]To obtain the 2.5th percentile, the statistical technique was modified to use the central 50% of the data for the Hoffmann plot. [b, c] To obtain the 2.5th and 97.5th percentiles, the statistical technique was modified to use the central 60% (instead of the usual 80%) of the data for the Hoffman plot.

RED CELL COUNT

Test	Age	Male			Female		
		n	$\times 10^6/\mu L$	$\times 10^{12}/L$	n	$\times 10^6/\mu L$	$\times 10^{12}/L$
1.	1 - 3d	76	4.2 - 5.5	4.2 - 5.5	76	3.4 - 5.4	3.4 - 5.4
	4 - 7d	49	3.9 - 5.4	3.9 - 5.4	39	3.5 - 5.5	3.5 - 5.5
	8 - 14d	60	3.4 - 5.1	3.4 - 5.1	69	3.2 - 5.0	3.2 - 5.0
	15 - 30d	168	3.1 - 4.6	3.1 - 4.6	116	3.1 - 4.6	3.1 - 4.6
	31 - 60d	562	2.9 - 3.9	2.9 - 3.9	419	2.9 - 4.1	2.9 - 4.1
	61 - 180d	1841	3.5 - 4.7	3.5 - 4.7	1363	3.4 - 4.6	3.4 - 4.6
	0.5 - <2y	8851	4.1 - 5.0	4.1 - 5.0	6934	4.1 - 4.9	4.1 - 4.9
	2 - <6y	11050	4.0 - 4.9	4.0 - 4.9	9752	4.0 - 4.9	4.0 - 4.9
	6 - <12y	7468	4.0 - 4.9	4.0 - 4.9	6804	4.0 - 4.9	4.0 - 4.9
	12 - <18y	5547	4.2 - 5.3	4.2 - 5.3	7977	4.0 - 4.9	4.0 - 4.9
	>18y	3171	3.8 - 5.4	3.8 - 5.4	8606	3.8 - 4.8	3.8 - 4.8
2.	1 - 3d	174	3.3 - 5.0	3.3 - 5.0	115	3.3 - 5.3	3.3 - 5.3
	4 - 7d	175	3.7 - 5.3	3.7 - 5.3	108	3.1 - 5.2	3.1 - 5.2
	8 - 14d	182	3.5 - 5.2	3.5 - 5.2	124	3.6 - 4.9	3.6 - 4.9
	15 - 30d	397	3.3 - 4.9	3.3 - 4.9	292	3.6 - 4.9	3.6 - 4.9
	31 - 60d	74	3.1 - 4.1	3.1 - 4.1	185	3.1 - 4.7	3.1 - 4.7
	61 - 180d	75	3.6 - 5.2	3.6 - 5.2	102	3.3 - 5.0	3.3 - 5.0
	0.5 - <2y	177	3.4 - 5.0	3.4 - 5.0	119	3.6 - 5.3	3.6 - 5.3
	2 - <6y	190	3.3[a] - 4.8	3.3[a] - 4.8	135	3.8[a] - 4.9	3.8[a] - 4.9
	6 - <12y	128	3.7[a] - 4.9	3.7[a] - 4.9	138	3.6[a] - 4.9	3.6[a] - 4.9
	12 - 18y	140	3.3[a] - 5.4	3.3[a] - 5.4	154	3.4[a] - 4.7	3.4[a] - 4.7
3.	1 - 14d	48	3.8 - 5.3	3.5 - 5.3	34	3.9 - 5.2	3.9 - 5.2
	15 - 30d	45	3.0 - 5.0	3.0 - 5.0	36	2.3 - 4.4	2.3 - 4.4
	31 - 60d	172	2.9 - 3.8	2.9 - 3.8	132	3.0 - 4.1	3.0 - 4.1
	61 - 180d	527	3.5 - 4.8	3.5 - 4.8	392	3.6 - 4.7	3.6 - 4.7
	0.5 - <2y	2056	4.1 - 6.0	4.1 - 6.0	1704	4.0 - 5.0	4.0 - 5.0
	2 - <6y	2403	4.1 - 5.0	4.1 - 5.0	2036	4.0 - 4.9	4.0 - 4.9
	6 - <12y	1931	3.9 - 5.0	3.9 - 5.0	1800	3.8 - 4.9	3.8 - 4.9
	12 - <18y	1731	3.8 - 5.3	3.8 - 5.3	2429	3.9 - 4.9	3.9 - 4.9
	>18y	1042	3.4 - 5.4	3.4 - 5.4	2505	3.7 - 4.8	3.7 - 4.8

Specimen Type:	1,2. Whole blood (K_3/EDTA anticoagulant) 3. Whole blood (K_2/EDTA anticoagulant)
Reference:	1, 2 Pediatric Reference Ranges, Eds. Soldin SJ, Brugnara C, et. al. 2nd Edition 1997 AACC Press. 3. Brugnara C. Manuscript in preparation.
Method(s):	1. Bayer H*3 (Bayer Diagnostics, Tarrytown, NY) 2. Coulter STKS (Beckman Coulter Inc., Brea, CA) 3. Bayer ADVIA 120 (Bayer Diagnostics, Tarrytown, NY)
Comments:	1,3. Data from outpatients. A computerized approach adapted from the Hoffmann technique was utilized to remove outliers and obtain the 2.5th and 97.5th percentiles. 2. Data from hospitalized patients (excluding hematology, oncology, and intensive care unit patients). A computerized approach adapted from the Hoffmann technique was utilized to remove outliers and obtain the 2.5th and 97.5th percentiles. [a]To obtain the 2.5th percentile, the statistical technique was modified to use the central 60% of the data for the Hoffmann plot.

RED CELL DISTRIBUTION WIDTH (RDW)

Test	Age	Male		Female	
		n	%	n	%
1.	1 - 3d	76	16.5 - 19.1	76	16.4 - 18.3
	4 - 7d	48	15.9 - 17.9	39	15.7 - 18.5
	8 - 14d	60	15.6 - 17.7	69	15.6 - 17.9
	15 - 30d	168	15.2 - 17.4	116	15.1 - 17.9
	31 - 60d	559	14.3 - 16.9	419	14.4 - 17.1
	61 - 180d	1834	12.6 - 15.5	1360	12.4 - 15.1
	0.5 - <2y	8828	13.1 - 15.6	6905	13.0 - 15.3
	2 - <6y	11126	12.9 - 15.0	9724	12.7 - 14.7
	6 - <12y	7449	12.7 - 14.6	6787	12.5 - 14.4
	12 - <18y	5542	12.7 - 14.6	7985	12.5 - 14.5
	> 18y	3162	12.8 - 15.2	8592	12.7 - 15.1
2.	1 - 3d	174	14.9 - 18.5	115	14.7 - 17.5
	4 - 7d	155	14.8 - 18.7	108	14.4 - 19.4
	8 - 14d	182	14.6 - 19.2	124	14.4 - 19.9
	15 - 30d	393	14.2 - 18.5	291	14.2 - 18.3
	31 - 60d	74	12.9 - 17.0	185	14.0 - 17.5
	61 - 180d	75	12.1 - 16.2	102	11.9 - 15.7
	0.5 - <2y	177	12.7 - 16.2	119	12.4 - 15.2
	2 - <6y	190	12.5 - 15.1	135	11.8 - 14.6
	6 - <12y	128	11.8 - 14.9	138	11.7 - 15.5
	12 - 18y	140	12.1 - 18.4	154	12.0 - 17.4
3.	1 - 14d	48	15.2 - 18.0	34	15.3 – 16.6
	15 - 30d	45	14.5 - 18.5	36	14.2 – 17.0
	31 - 60d	169	13.8 – 16.3	132	14.0 – 16.4
	61 - 180d	526	12.2 – 15.0	388	12.1 – 14.5
	0.5 - <2y	2055	12.7 – 15.0	1700	12.6 – 14.7
	2 - <6y	2396	12.5 – 14.3	2036	12.3 – 14.3
	6 - <12y	1922	12.2 – 14.2	1794	12.2 – 14.5
	12 - <18y	1752	12.3 – 14.7	2419	12.1 – 14.4
	>18y	1040	12.4 – 15.0	2503	12.4 – 15.3

Specimen Type:	1,2. Whole blood (K$_3$/EDTA anticoagulant)
	3. Whole blood (K$_2$/EDTA anticoagulant)
Reference:	1, 2 Pediatric Reference Ranges, Eds. Soldin SJ, Brugnara C, et. al. 2nd Edition 1997 AACC Press.
	3. Brugnara C. Manuscript in preparation.
Method(s):	1. Bayer H*3 (Bayer Diagnostics, Tarrytown, NY)
	2. Coulter STKS (Beckman Coulter Inc., Brea, CA)
	3. Bayer ADVIA 120 (Bayer Diagnostics, Tarrytown, NY)
Comments:	1,3. Data from outpatients. A computerized approach adapted from the Hoffmann technique was utilized to remove outliers and obtain the 2.5th and 97.5th percentiles.
	2. Data from hospitalized patients (excluding hematology, oncology, and intensive care unit patients). A computerized approach adapted from the Hoffmann technique was utilized to remove outliers and obtain the 2.5th and 97.5th percentiles.

RETICULOCYTE COUNT (ABSOLUTE)

		Male			Female		
Test	Age	n	$\times 10^3$ /μL	$\times 10^9$/L	n	$\times 10^3$ /μL	$\times 10^9$/L
1.	1 - <6mo	66	37 - 104	37 - 104	24	52 - 120	52 - 120
	6mo - <2y	68	29 - 89	29 - 89	78	35 - 92	35 - 92
	2 - <6y	126	29 - 80	29 - 80	92	43 - 83	43 - 83
	6 - <12y	129	39 - 106	39 - 106	115	37 - 93	37 - 93
	12 - <18y	204	39 - 100	39 - 100	216	40 - 102	40 - 102
	>18y	213	43 - 85	43 - 85	392	46 - 102	46 - 102

Specimen Type:	Whole blood (K$_2$/EDTA anticoagulant)
Reference:	Brugnara C. Manuscript in preparation.
Method(s):	Bayer ADVIA 120 (Bayer Diagnostics, Tarrytown, NY)
Comments:	Data from outpatients. A computerized approach adapted from the Hoffmann technique was utilized to remove outliers and obtain the 2.5th and 97.5th percentiles.

RETICULOCYTE COUNT (RELATIVE)

Test	Age	Male			Female		
		n	%	Number Fraction	n	%	Number Fraction
1.	1 - 3d	22	2.2 - 4.8	.022 - .048	26	2.1 - 3.7	.021 - .037
	4 - 30d	58	0.4 - 2.7	.004 - .027	29	0.4 - 2.0	.004 - .020
	31 - 60d	67	0.9 - 3.8	.009 - .038	34	1.5 - 3.2	.015 - .032
	61 - 180d	138	0.9 - 3.1	.009 - .031	98	1.1 - 2.9	.011 - .029
	0.5 - <2y	602	0.8 - 2.0	.008 - .020	439	0.9 - 2.0	.009 - .020
	2 - <6y	966	0.8 - 2.0	.008 - .020	770	0.8 - 2.1	.008 - .021
	6 - <12y	688	0.7 - 2.2	.007 - .022	570	0.8 - 2.8	.008 - .028
	12 - 18y	480	0.8 - 2.2	.008 - .022	558	0.8 - 2.2	.008 - .022

Specimen Type:	Whole blood (K$_3$/EDTA anticoagulant)
Reference:	Pediatric Reference Ranges, Eds. Soldin SJ, Brugnara C, et. al. 2nd Edition 1997 AACC Press.
Method(s):	Bayer H*3 (Bayer Diagnostics, Tarrytown, NY)
Comments:	Data from outpatients. A computerized approach adapted from the Hoffmann technique was utilized to remove outliers and obtain the 2.5th and 97.5th percentiles.

WHITE CELL COUNT

Test	Age	Male			Female		
		n	$\times 10^3/\mu L$	$\times 10^9/L$	n	$\times 10^3/\mu L$	$\times 10^9/L$
1.	1 - 3d	76	6.8 – 13.3	6.8 - 13.3	76	8.0 - 14.3	8.0 - 14.3
	4 - 7d	48	8.3 – 14.1	8.3 - 14.1	39	8.8 - 14.8	8.8 - 14.8
	8 - 14d	59	8.2 – 14.4	8.2 - 14.4	68	8.4 - 15.4	8.4 - 15.4
	15 - 30d	167	7.4 – 14.6	7.4 - 14.6	115	8.3 - 14.7	8.3 - 14.7
	31 - 60d	560	6.7 – 14.2	6.7 - 14.2	415	7.0 - 15.1	7.0 - 15.1
	61 - 180d	1832	6.9 – 15.7	6.9 - 15.7	1359	6.8 - 16.0	6.8 - 16.0
	0.5 - <2y	8751	6.2 – 14.5	6.2 - 14.5	6829	6.4 - 15.0	6.4 - 15.0
	2 - <6y	11056	5.3 – 11.5	5.3 - 11.5	9675	5.3 - 11.5	5.3 - 11.5
	6 - <12y	7431	4.5 – 10.5	4.5 - 10.5	6718	4.7 - 10.3	4.7 - 10.3
	12 - <18y	5519	4.5 – 10.0	4.5 - 10.0	7971	4.8 - 10.1	4.8 - 10.1
	> 18y	3133	4.4 – 10.2	4.4 - 10.2	8571	4.9 - 10.0	4.9 - 10.0
2.	1 - 3d	174	5.5 – 15.0	5.5 - 15.0	115	8.4 - 16.6	8.4 - 16.6
	4 - 7d	175	6.2 – 13.0	6.2 - 13.0	108	7.9 - 16.0	7.9 - 16.0
	8 - 14d	182	7.8[a] – 19.3[b]	9.0 - 20.7	124	7.3[a] - 16.5[b]	9.2 - 17.8
	15 - 30d	369	7.2[a] – 19.9[b]	9.0 - 22.1	292	7.2[a] - 18.4[b]	9.1 - 19.6
	31 - 60d	392	7.4 – 14.3	7.4 - 14.3	185	8.2 - 16.3	8.2 - 16.3
	61 - 180d	75	8.3 – 15.9	8.3 - 15.9	102	7.9 - 13.4	7.9 - 13.4
	0.5 - <2y	177	7.8 – 14.8	7.8 - 14.8	119	6.3 - 12.6	6.3 - 12.6
	2 - <6y	190	5.0 – 13.2	5.0 - 13.2	135	6.4 - 11.1	6.4 - 11.1
	6 - <12y	128	5.0 – 11.8	5.0 - 11.8	138	4.8 - 10.7	4.8 - 10.7
	12 - <18y	140	5.1 – 15.5	5.1 - 15.5	154	4.9 - 9.1	4.9 - 9.1
3.	1 - 14d	47	8.6 – 14.9	8.6 - 14.9	34	8.3 - 17.6	8.3 - 17.6
	15 - 30d	45	7.4 – 13.3	7.4 - 13.3	36	6.9 - 15.0	6.9 - 15.0
	31 - 60d	169	6.0 – 13.7	6.0 - 13.7	131	6.1 - 13.8	6.1 - 13.8
	61 - 180d	526	6.6 – 15.6	6.6 - 15.6	391	6.8 - 16.2	6.8 - 16.2
	0.5 - <2y	2042	6.3 – 15.4	6.3 - 15.4	1694	6.4 - 15.5	6.4 - 15.5
	2 - <6y	2392	5.5 – 12.3	5.5 - 12.3	2024	5.5 - 12.5	5.5 - 12.5
	6 - <12y	1911	4.7 – 11.3	4.7 - 11.3	1791	4.9 - 11.4	4.9 - 11.4
	12 - <18y	1756	4.4 – 10.5	4.4 - 10.5	2416	4.9 - 10.4	4.9 - 10.4
	>18y	1027	4.3 – 10.4	4.3 - 10.4	2500	4.9 - 10.7	4.9 - 10.7

Specimen Type:	1,2.	Whole blood (K_3/EDTA anticoagulant)
	3.	Whole blood (K_2/EDTA anticoagulant)
Reference:	1, 2	Pediatric Reference Ranges, Eds. Soldin SJ, Brugnara C, et. al. 2nd Edition 1997 AACC Press.
	3.	Brugnara C. Manuscript in preparation.
Method(s):	1.	Bayer H*3 (Bayer Diagnostics, Tarrytown, NY)
	2.	Coulter STKS (Beckman Coulter Inc., Brea, CA)
	3.	Bayer ADVIA 120 (Bayer Diagnostics, Tarrytown, NY)
Comments:	1,3.	Data from outpatients. A computerized approach adapted from the Hoffmann technique was utilized to remove outliers and obtain the 2.5th and 97.5th percentiles.
	2.	Data from hospitalized patients (excluding hematology, oncology, and intensive care unit patients). A computerized approach adapted from the Hoffmann technique was utilized to remove outliers and obtain the 2.5th and 97.5th percentiles. To obtain the 2.5th percentile, the statistical technique was modified to use the central 60% of the data for the Hoffmann plot.
		[a]Central 80% used for 2.5th percentile [b]Central 50% used for 97.5th percentile